Drugs and the Elderly

DRUGS
AND THE
ELDERLY

Clinical, Social, and Policy Perspectives

::

Helene Levens Lipton, Ph.D.
Philip R. Lee, M.D.

with contributions by
Mark S. Freeland, Ph.D.

::

Stanford University Press :: Stanford, California

1988

Stanford University Press
Stanford, California

© 1988 by the Board of Trustees of the
Leland Stanford Junior University

Printed and bound by CPI Group (UK) Ltd,
Croydon, CR0 4YY

CIP data are at the end of the book

Acknowledgments

There are many people without whose encouragement and support this work would never have been completed. They fully deserve to share in any accolades this book may be awarded, but they should shoulder no blame for any errors, omissions, or misrepresentations we may have made. It is exceedingly difficult to single out everyone who has contributed to this volume over the years. But we are particularly grateful to the following individuals and organizations: Milton Silverman, Ph.D., and Mia Lydecker for the wisdom that comes from a life-long commitment to the study of prescription drugs and drug policies and for their work in this field; Harold Luft, Ph.D., Institute for Health Policy Studies, University of California at San Francisco (UCSF), for his thorough and painstaking reviews of the entire manuscript (on multiple occasions), his constructive criticisms, and brilliant ideas; our colleagues in the Division of Clinical Pharmacy, School of Pharmacy, at UCSF—Toby Herfindal (Pharm.D., M.P.H.), Ron Finley (B.S. Pharm.), and Gary McCart (Pharm.D.)—whose enormous expertise helped shape our knowledge and understanding of drug therapy in the elderly in all of its complexities and challenges; Bonnie L. Svarstad, Ph.D., University of Wisconsin (Madison), for sharing with us her scholarly and insightful ideas in research methodology—and for helping us to define not only what is known but also what needs to be known; Jerry Avorn, M.D., Harvard Medical School, for his invaluable counsel, information, and advice all along the way in areas as diverse as drug pharmacokinetics and drug policy; John Virts, Ph.D., Eli Lilly Company, for his invaluable information on the drug industry's perspectives; Robert Temple, M.D., Food and Drug Administration, for his help in teaching us the nature and complexities of the drug regulatory process; Nelda McCall, SRI International, for her informative and thoughtful review and critique of the policy section of the manuscript; Joel Rotenberg, for his excellent editorial assistance, his unbelievable word processing skills, and his endurance; Lynn Goldman, for her excellent editorial assistance, and Pat Coray, for her help in preparing the manuscript; Eunice Chee, Institute for Health Policy Studies, UCSF, for coordinating the production of multiple drafts of the manuscript and for her soothing calm and sound counsel in calamitous times; Grant Barnes and Clare Novak at Stanford University Press, for their confidence in us and for their belief in the value of our work; Jean Nattkemper, our manuscript editor, for her outstanding editorial skills and inordinate good cheer; and the Administration on Aging, U.S. Department of Health and Human Services, for its financial support, which gave us the impetus to begin and continue this work.

And finally, a special and heartfelt thanks goes to our families—especially Andrew, Josh, and Shira Lipton, Mynnye Levens, and Carroll Estes—for their encouragement, patience, and contributions throughout these many years. Words can never fully describe how much they are cherished for the love and support they showed throughout this entire enterprise.

We are indeed blessed to have had help from such valued colleagues, co-workers, friends, and family.

H.L.L.
P.R.L.

San Francisco

Contents

Foreword

Jere E. Goyan

It comes as a bit of a shock to realize that the flamboyant, fiery, fox-trotting "bobcats" and "flappers" of the 1920s—immortalized by F. Scott Fitzgerald as the "lost generation"—have crossed an unmarked border and entered a realm deemed by some (not them) to be the "golden years," and by others to be the "declining years." With that eventful passage came the acquisition of a series of unwanted labels, including "senior citizens," "the aged," "the elderly," and "the old folks." Although this generation had been tagged according to age before—they were "children," then "youths," and then "adults"—these new labels have an entirely different connotation. To the patronizing society that has created them, they mean people who are to be cherished but are no longer "productive." To most who wear the labels, however, they are merely cause for frustration.

It is probable that the elderly of the nation would agree with the sentiment of the title of a recent book, "The Golden Years Are a Crock," especially as far as their health was concerned. In regard to health, the elderly have again become a "lost generation," lost this time through oversight. Until fairly recently, science has devoted very little energy to unraveling the mysteries of aging, especially as they relate to drug therapy. What science knew came primarily in the form of statistics that simplistically profiled the elderly as persons who consumed more health care services, took more drugs, and were more prone to chronic illness than the young. It was an uninterested view at best, derived from the flawed assumption that, aside from certain

JERE E. GOYAN, Ph.D., is Dean of the School of Pharmacy at the University of California, San Francisco. He was Commissioner of the Food and Drug Administration from 1979 to 1981.

obvious differences, an elderly person was simply a slowed-down version of someone younger. It is not surprising, therefore, that for years many problems uniquely afflicting the elderly, including an increased rate of iatrogenic illness and adverse effects from prescription and nonprescription drugs, went unnoticed or were attributed to other factors.

The elderly were the victims of timing as well as time. Only recently have adverse reactions to drugs—including undesired reactions between two or more drugs—become well documented and routinely recognized. As late as the 1970s, it was possible to find physicians who maintained that they had never seen an adverse drug reaction in any patient, young or old. Yet, because statistics make it clear that such effects were, in fact, taking place, it is probable that prescribers did indeed see them, but attributed what they saw to other causes.

The elderly are even overlooked by the system whereby new drugs are approved. In 1962, the Food, Drug, and Cosmetic Act was amended to require that a drug be effective (as well as safe) for the malady it was claimed to treat before it could be approved for marketing by the Food and Drug Administration. However, studies demonstrating safety and efficacy were, for the most part, limited to people between the ages of 20 and 60, despite the fact that significant portions of our population are younger or older. However, as the pediatrician Harry Shirkey pointed out a number of years ago, children are not simply miniature adults in the way their bodies handle drugs. He referred to them as "therapeutic orphans," because so few drugs had been studied in children. More recently, a similar criticism has been voiced on behalf of the elderly. Many experts are now calling for a requirement that a drug be tested for safety and efficacy in the elderly before being approved.

Public policymakers have also been remiss in addressing fully the elderly's drug therapy needs. Although the elderly pay more per capita for drugs than do members of any other age group, Medicare does not cover out-of-hospital prescription drug costs. For millions of elderly, soaring drug costs are a severe problem.

Until recently, the elderly were also overlooked in terms of research conducted about their drug needs. Studies in this area did not even appear on the agendas of the major federal agencies funding research. However, in the past few years, there have been a growing number of studies on the elderly, especially related to their use of drugs. Aside from epidemiological studies regarding drug utilization, researchers have discovered that the metabolic rate for many drugs in the elderly may be one-half to two-thirds the rate of younger adults. Similarly, many drugs may be excreted far more slowly. Thus, the elderly may have been grossly overdosed in certain instances and unnecessarily exposed to adverse drug effects. Many more studies are needed, especially in the areas of dosing and frequency of administration, both before drugs are approved for marketing and after marketing. In addition, research findings need to be incorporated into the professional education of pharmacists and physicians.

The authors of this book have done an outstanding job, not only in sorting through the reams of data that have been generated in the past few years, but in evaluating them and bringing them together in a readable form. In this comprehensive book, geriatric drug use is studied in all of its many dimensions, ranging from the pharmacokinetic and pharmacodynamic aspects of drug use and misuse to physician prescribing and drug costs. Particularly notable are the strategies that the authors propose for reducing inappropriate prescribing by physicians and noncompliance among their aged patients, and the broad-based and detailed action agenda, designed to alleviate the problems that have been identified. The book will be valuable for health policymakers; for instructors, particularly in pharmacy, medicine, dentistry, and nursing; for practitioners; for social and behavioral scientists interested in geriatrics; and for consumers seeking a better understanding of the issues related to drugs and the elderly.

In the past, many of us have "cursed the darkness" surrounding drug use in the elderly. We are all indebted to the authors of this book for lighting more than the first candle. This, and perhaps other efforts of a similar nature, can help lead us to enlightened drug therapy so that the older generation, of which we will all one day be members, will no longer be "lost."

Preface

When we think of the "drug problem" in the United States, the image of the elderly is not the first to come to mind. Yet the use and misuse of prescription drugs by older people is a subject of increasing concern. This book responds to five critical issues facing Americans: the rapid growth of the elderly population—those people 65 years of age or older; widespread problems of drug misuse among the elderly; the elderly's need to receive more detailed information about their drugs; inappropriate prescribing by physicians; and the failure of researchers, physicians, pharmacists, drug manufacturers, and health policymakers to address adequately the elderly's problems in using prescription drugs.

In discussions about "the elderly," we often assume that they are a homogeneous group, but the facts show quite the contrary. The elderly population is made up of subgroups, which vary with respect to income, social class, health status, living arrangements, and marital status. Such subgroups include the healthy elderly, who are more likely to be married and belong to the middle or upper class; the terminally ill elderly, who are afflicted with chronic pain and are unable to secure adequate relief; the frail noninstitutionalized elderly, who take multiple medications and may suffer adverse drug reactions; the chronically ill elderly, who reside both in nursing homes and hospitals and who are prescribed a large number of drugs concurrently; the lonely impoverished female elderly, many of whom routinely receive mood-altering medications to relieve problems primarily social in origin; and the low-income elderly, who cannot afford to pay the rising prices for prescription drugs. All of these groups will be addressed in our book.

In the past fifty years, more and more prescription drugs have been developed and marketed for an ever-widening range of diseases. The increase in the variety and quantity of drugs, the knowledge of their benefits, and the widespread clinical use of drugs have far outdistanced our understanding of the problems associated with their use. Inadequate knowledge about drug use is more dangerous in relation to the elderly, because aged people become ill more often, suffer more from chronic conditions that are treatable with drugs, and are prescribed more drugs than are younger adults or children. Because of the sheer number of drugs prescribed, the elderly often have difficulty taking their drugs as indicated—that is, they have a problem with drug compliance. Moreover, because the elderly respond to drugs differently than do younger people, they face a greater likelihood of adverse drug reactions. The elderly who use prescription drugs, particularly those who are poor but ineligible for Medicaid, face the additional problems of rising drug prices.

The problems intensify because of the increase in the number of elderly. The rapid growth of the elderly population has led many commentators to label the United States an "aging society." The number of elderly has risen swiftly since the turn of the century and has doubled since 1950, reaching 28 million in 1984. The fastest growing group in the population is made up of those age 85 years and over; they have quadrupled since 1950, and in 1984 numbered 2.6 million (Siegel & Taeuber 1986). By 1990 the number of people 65 years of age or older will increase to 32.4 million, or 12.6 percent of the population. By the year 2030, when most of the baby boom generation will have reached age 65 years or older, the elderly will number 55 million, or 18.3 percent of the population (Wade 1985).

The 11 percent of Americans who were elderly in 1980 received almost 30 percent of all prescription drugs used in this country. Among the elderly who were not in hospitals or nursing homes, 85 percent used drugs on a regular basis: 67 percent took at least one drug daily, and 25 percent took three or more drugs daily. The corresponding figures for younger persons were 43 percent and 9 percent (American Association of Retired Persons 1984). Because noninstitutionalized elderly use numerous nonprescription, or over-the-counter, drugs in addition to prescription drugs, there is the potential for drug-drug interactions that the patient does not recognize as drug-related. This poses a problem for physicians who care for elderly patients.

Drugs are used in response to chronic illness, which becomes more common with age and is a major cause of disability among the elderly. Forty-four percent have arthritis, 38 percent have hypertension, 28 percent have hearing impairments, and 27 percent have heart conditions (National Center for Health Statistics & Jack 1981). Furthermore, increasing numbers of elderly have more than one chronic condition (Rice & LaPlante 1986). The number of chronically ill, functionally disabled elderly who reside in nursing homes is steadily growing, and their per capita use of drugs is extremely high. Risks involving inappropriate use and adverse drug reactions increase in tandem. The problem is compounded by the low payments made by Medicaid for nursing home care for the elderly.

Although drugs are used by so many of the elderly, we still lack information on many issues concerning drug use and the aged. A great deal is now known about patient noncompliance with drug therapy. Not as much is known about the reasons and remedies for inappropriate physician prescribing. Some, but not enough, study has been devoted to examining the drug costs borne by the elderly, particularly those who are poor and those hovering just above the poverty threshold. Nor do we fully appreciate the difficult and dangerous decisions many elderly make as a direct consequence of high prescription drug costs—tragic choices not to take life-saving drugs or to redirect limited financial resources to pay for drugs in lieu of other essentials, such as food and shelter.

In the years ahead, difficult decisions must be made regarding how to protect the elderly from rising drug costs while simultaneously improving the quality and economy of geriatric drug prescribing and use. We hope that this book will provide policymakers, health professionals, and the public with a useful framework for thinking about these issues and achieving these objectives.

Drugs and the Aging Person

CHAPTER ONE

Drug Therapy for the Elderly: The Importance of Biological Changes with Age

Introduction

Because the number of elderly persons is growing, there is increased attention on the need for rational prescribing by physicians and appropriate drug use by aged patients. The elderly's burden of chronic illness and disability, their frequent use of drugs, the costs of drug treatment, and the benefits and risks of drug therapy are attracting considerable notice in the medical literature (Rowe 1977; Vestal 1978; Schmucker 1979, 1984; Ouslander 1981; Greenblatt, Sellers & Shader 1982; Conrad & Bressler 1982; Becker & Cohen 1984; Lamy 1984; Kelly 1986). Growing evidence indicates, however, that in the absence of disease many of the body's organ systems maintain normal function into old age (Rodeheffer et al. 1984; Shibaski et al. 1984). Evidence also indicates that an individual's basic personality traits change little with age (McCrae & Costa 1984). Williams (1986) has noted the body's plasticity (ability to improve or restore function) despite aging. Thus, even though the elderly face disease-related problems, many myths about aging as a period of inevitable physical and mental decline are fast disappearing.

Advances in therapeutics during the past fifty years have brought great benefits. Almost all areas of drug therapy have been touched by these advances. Yet with the benefits have come problems, caused by the marketing of drugs of questionable efficacy by industry, irrational prescribing by physicians, inappropriate dispensing by pharmacists, and misuse of drugs and adverse drug reactions among the elderly.

Biological, psychological, and social changes that occur with age may affect the elderly's response to prescription drugs. Although we recognize the importance of social and psychological factors affecting use of and response to drugs, because of the lack of research in this area we will emphasize the biological factors. These include both the biological changes that accompany aging and those that result from disease. Before proceeding to these issues, however, we shall first discuss briefly the physician's role in drug treatment.

Clinical Assessment: The First Step in Drug Treatment

The first step in drug treatment is a careful clinical assessment by the patient's physician of the patient's history, present illness, and physical and psychosocial status. Using this assessment, the physician identifies the origins of the patient's symptoms as accurately as possible and determines whether they can be improved by or are related to drug therapy. If the patient's symptoms are related to drug therapy, the physician should modify the dosage or discontinue use of the offending drug. If a drug or drugs are needed, the physician must make a careful appraisal of the factors affecting the patient's response to drugs.

The physician's clinical assessment of the elderly patient is complicated by the altered presentation of a variety of common diseases and the presence of multiple chronic conditions affecting several organ systems (Lamy 1984). Not only do particular diseases alter the body's response to drugs, but diseases may present themselves differently in the elderly (Conrad & Bressler 1982). Confusion, falls, and urinary incontinence may be viewed as inevitable consequences of aging when, in fact, they may represent symptoms of treatable systemic illnesses or adverse drug reactions (Steel 1978; Ouslander 1981). Painless myocardial infarction, sepsis without fever, and pneumonia presenting as confusion are among the common age-related differences in presentation of illness (Rowe 1977). Often, potentially treatable conditions are not recognized by physicians and other health professionals (Brocklehurst et al. 1978; Williams et al. 1973). The implications of this problem for the elderly are serious: unrecognized conditions remain untreated. If misinterpreted, the illnesses may be treated with inappropriate drug therapy, which can exacerbate the underlying condition or affect the outcome of therapy for other illnesses treated simultaneously.

When pharmacological treatment is necessary, the prescribing physician may be uncertain about the dosage to be prescribed for an elderly patient. Some physicians recommend doses that are 30 to 50 percent of those used for younger adults, particularly for psychotropic drugs (Thompson, Moran & Nies 1983). Although this may be appropriate, it is preferable to calculate the dose carefully and, when possible, monitor drug concentrations in the blood. It is also important that the physician discuss the proposed drug treatment with the patient and, if necessary, with the patient's family. This discussion should include information on all prescriptions used outside the hospital or nursing home. Ideally, verbal instruction should be supplemented with written instruction provided by the physician and the pharmacist.

In any drug therapy it is essential that the physician have a system for carefully monitoring the drug's effects. Monitoring, especially for drugs used on a long-term basis, can often be done effectively in close collaboration with the pharmacist and the patient. Careful monitoring can also include discontinuing the drug to observe whether or not continued treatment is necessary (Everitt & Avorn 1986).

Assessing Altered Drug Effects in the Elderly

To understand the altered response to drugs in old age, it is helpful to view aging from a biopsychosocial perspective and not merely from a biological or biomedical perspective (Engel 1977; Grody & Sobel 1979; Becker & Cohen 1984). Becker and Cohen have identified three types of changes that may affect the functional status of the elderly: biological (e.g., gradual decline in physiological reserves of most organ systems), psychological (e.g., changes in perceptual and cognitive capabilities), and social (e.g., loss of social support). All of these factors must also be considered in evaluating the elderly patient's response to drugs.

One biopsychosocial dimension of aging is increased differentiation among individuals; there is greater heterogeneity among the elderly than among the young (Becker & Cohen 1984). Therefore, the elderly show more variability in their response to drugs. Age itself is a factor in an individual's response to drugs: at age 85 the response may be quite different from what it was at age 75 or 65.

Another factor to be considered in assessing drug effects is altered response to stress with age. In the elderly the reserve capacity of the body and the speed of response of various organ systems under stress are decreased in many body functions. These changes may be caused by chronic disease or, in some cases, by the aging process itself. Whatever the cause, they make an elderly patient under stress more sensitive to the effects of a variety of drugs, particularly those affecting the cardiovascular system, the brain, and the kidneys (e.g., antihypertensives, diuretics, sedative-hypnotics, tranquilizers, and antipsychotics).

Altered Biological Response to Drugs with Aging

Age-related biological changes that affect the elderly's response to drugs include differences in the distribution, metabolism, and excretion of drugs and differences in the effects of drugs at the cellular level. Two quite different hypotheses have been developed to explain these age-related changes (Greenblatt, Sellers & Shader 1982; Schmucker 1984). Some investigators postulate that an alteration in receptor site sensitivity at the cellular level may account for the elderly's enhanced or diminished response to many drugs (pharmacodynamic hypothesis). A drug acts at the cellular level by attaching to receptor molecules that are involved in controlling the normal chemical reactions within the cell. Changes at the site of drug action—either a change in the number of receptors on the cell or changes in the intracellular processes after the initial drug-receptor interaction—occur with age and may affect the elderly patient's response to drugs (Rowe 1977; Greenblatt, Sellers & Shader 1982). Because of such changes, a given concentration of a drug will produce a greater or lesser reaction in an elderly person than in a younger person. Information on receptor site processes is scarce, but clinical observations suggest the existence of such a mechanism to account for drug effects that are independent of drug absorption, metabolism, distribution, and excretion (Shepherd 1977; Reidenberg et al. 1978).

There is relatively little empirical evidence to support the pharmacodynamic hypothesis, although it remains a possibility. The more widely accepted view is that age-dependent changes in drug disposition due to changes in drug absorption, metabolism, distribution, or excretion are largely responsible for enhanced drug sensitivity in the elderly (pharmacokinetic hypothesis).

Drug Absorption

Most drugs are taken by mouth and absorbed into the body through the gastrointestinal tract. Although there has been much speculation about altered drug absorption from the gastrointestinal tract into the bloodstream, there is no firm evidence that drug absorption is impaired in old age (Triggs & Nation 1975; Ouslander 1981; Greenblatt, Sellers & Shader 1982). An important factor affecting the absorption of drugs at all ages is interaction with foods. The presence of food in the gastrointestinal tract may affect absorption of a drug directly or through effects on motility in the gut. Food may decrease, delay, or, in some cases, enhance absorption of a drug. The absorption of antibiotics such as ampicillin, tetracycline, and penicillin G may be decreased or delayed when taken with meals (Krondl 1970). Tetracycline absorption may also be reduced if taken with antacids or dairy products. For many drug products—for example, aspirin—absorption is prolonged by food, but the extent of absorption is not reduced (Goodman & Gilman 1970). Drugs that are often absorbed better when taken with food include the antihypertensives hydralazine and propranolol. Food may also be recommended for its capacity to prevent gastric irritation caused by drugs (e.g., aspirin).

Thus, it is important for physicians, in prescribing drugs, and pharmacists, in dispensing them, to give elderly patients specific information on when to take a drug in relation to meals. Because many patients have difficulty in remembering such details, printed information is a useful supplement to verbal instructions.

Not only may the absorption of drugs be affected by meals, but drugs may also lead to a variety of nutritional problems that can have additional effects on a patient's response to a drug. Most drug-food interactions that might lead to nutritional deficiencies in elderly patients are preventable if risk factors are recognized and appropriate actions taken. Risk factors include multiple medications, long-term drug therapy, chronic disease, low income, poor nutritional habits, and lack of knowledge of the adverse nutritional effects of drugs by physicians, pharmacists, and nurses. We shall have more to say about the relationship between nutrition and drug use in a subsequent section of this chapter.

Drug Metabolism

A drug taken by mouth is absorbed into the bloodstream and passes first into the liver, where drug metabolism usually takes place. Factors controlling metabolism include liver blood flow, genetic factors (some individuals lack the enzymes necessary to metabolize particular drugs), and the liver enzyme systems. Although age does not alter genetic factors, it can affect both liver blood flow and the rate at which drugs are metabolized in the liver (Bender 1965; Vestal et al. 1979). Thus, the body's capacity to metabolize drugs may be altered (Triggs & Nation 1975; Richey & Bender 1977; Greenblatt, Sellers & Shader 1982).

Changes in liver enzymes caused by age vary. With advancing age, decreased clearance for drugs such as diazepam, chlordiazepoxide, theophylline, and nortriptyline has been observed. However, there is no decrease in clearance for other drugs, such as the benzodiazepines lorazepam and oxazepam (Kelly 1986).

Although the liver's capacity to metabolize and clear drugs changes in old age, it is not easy to predict how an individual patient may be affected. Furthermore, the patient may be given a drug in a number of ways: by mouth, by intramuscular injection, or by intravenous injection. Drugs given intravenously may reach cell receptors without passing through the liver. In addition, the patient may be a heavy drinker of alcohol, a cigarette smoker, or a heavy coffee drinker—all factors that may directly or indirectly affect the metabolism of the drug in the liver.

Drug Distribution

Following absorption from the gastrointestinal tract and passage through the liver, drugs or their metabolic products are distributed to receptor sites on cells throughout the body. Drug distribution is affected primarily by body composition (lean body mass, body water, adipose tissue mass) and the extent to which a drug is bound by plasma proteins, particularly albumin. Body composition of individuals may differ because of age or gender (women have a higher percentage of adipose tissue), and the body composition of an individual may change because of malnutrition or diseases associated with weight loss.

Changes in body composition that accompany aging, particularly the proportion of fat in relation to other tissue, may influence drug distribution. In the elderly, in general, fat tissue mass increases and lean body mass decreases in relation to total body weight. Total body water is 10 to 15 percent less and body fat 10 to 20 percent greater in the elderly than in younger subjects (Vestal et al. 1978). Thus, actual lean body mass is reduced as a proportion of total body weight. By age 65 years, the average man has 12 kilograms less and the average woman 5 kilograms less lean body mass than the average middle-aged man or woman. The effects of proportion of lean body mass and fatty tissue on the body's response to a drug depend on the drug's solubility in water and fat.

In general, drugs distributed mainly in body water or lean body mass have higher blood levels if the dose is based only on body weight or surface area, whereas fat-soluble (lipid-soluble) drugs are more extensively distributed and thus have lower blood levels. Studies of the distribution of alcohol, which is water-soluble when given intravenously, reveal no change in the rate of elimination by the kidneys in the elderly when compared with younger adults. However, significantly higher peak blood levels of alcohol are found in the elderly, attributable to the small volume of body water and lean body mass (Vestal et al. 1977). Conversely, fat-soluble drugs, such as diazepam and lidocaine, may be more widely distributed in the elderly because of increase in fatty tissue relative to total body weight. Fat-soluble drugs thus have a lower concentration at the site of action in the elderly than in younger adults (Greenblatt, Sellers & Shader 1982). However, the effects of these drugs may be altered because they are distributed in fatty tissues and may be released gradually to the bloodstream.

In addition to body composition, drug distribution is affected by the extent to which the drug is bound to plasma proteins, particularly albumin. (A drug that is not bound to plasma proteins is the active form of the drug.) A decline in the concentration of plasma proteins has been consistently observed among the elderly. This reduction is even more marked in the elderly who have chronic diseases, especially diseases associated with malnutrition. Drugs that are highly bound to plasma proteins are likely to cause problems if this fact is not considered. For example, drugs such as propranolol, an antihypertensive, and warfarin, an anticoagulant, might cause adverse reactions in the elderly because they are highly bound to serum albumin. Because of the aged person's lower levels of serum albumin, more unbound active drug is distributed to cellular receptor sites (Irvine et al. 1974; Wallace, Whiting & Runcie 1976; Rowe 1977).

Drug Excretion

The role of the kidneys in drug clearance is less complex and better understood than is drug metabolism in the liver. However, it is not easy to separate changes in the kidneys caused by aging from those caused by disease. Until very recently it was widely believed that kidney function declines progressively with age, with a mean reduction of 35 percent in the kidney's filtering capacity in the elderly compared with middle-aged and younger adults (Rowe et al. 1976a, 1976b; Friedman et al. 1972; Epstein 1979). For drugs in which total clearance from the body is accomplished partly or entirely by excretion of the intact drug by the kidneys (e.g., penicillin), renal clearance declines approximately in proportion to the decline in the filtering capacity (measured as glomerular filtration rate).

In a study of the effects of aging on glomerular filtration rate among healthy volunteers of the Baltimore Study on Aging, Lindeman, Tobin, and Shock (1985) reported that, although there is a mean decline of 0.75 mgm/ml/m² in creatinine clearance per year in elderly subjects, there is substantial variability. No change with aging was found in about 30 percent of the volunteers, an actual increase in about 5 percent, and a variable decline in the remaining 65 percent. The finding is of great clinical relevance. It means that the clinician can no longer rely exclusively on standard formulas to calculate glomerular filtration rate but must, instead, determine renal function and/or determine drug concentrations in the blood.

The clearance of drugs that achieve effects through the drug's active metabolites rather than the intact drug will also be altered when these metabolites are cleared by the kidneys. These include the tranquilizer diazepam and the sedative-hypnotic flurazepam (Greenblatt, Sellers & Shader 1982).

Adverse Drug Reactions

What Is an Adverse Drug Reaction?

An adverse drug reaction can be defined simply as any harmful or unwanted effect caused by a drug taken in its regular dosage. An adverse drug reaction is marked by the following characteristics:

☐ It is adverse—noxious, untoward, or pathological.

☐ It is unintended and not a goal of treatment.

☐ It results from the administration of a normal dosage of a legally available drug prescribed for an appropriate medical indication.

☐ It is not mild or trivial in degree.

Three general types of adverse drug reactions have been identified: (1) side effects, which occur quite predictably (e.g., constipation is often a side effect of morphine given to control severe pain); (2) hypersensitivity or allergic reactions, which occur only in persons allergic to a particular drug and which may be mild (e.g., itching of the skin), very severe (anaphylactic reaction), or even fatal; (3) toxic reactions, which usually result from drug overdose or poisoning, but may occur in the elderly because of increased sensitivity to a normal dose due to diminished kidney function, decreased body water, or other biological changes accompanying age.

Adverse Drug Reactions Among the Elderly

Although drugs in general are remarkably nontoxic, the elderly are more likely to suffer adverse drug reactions than are patients under 65 years of age. There are three primary reasons for this: (1) Biological changes with aging affect the individual's response to drugs; (2) The burden of chronic illness results in the prescription of multiple drugs, particularly in hospitals and nursing homes; (3) Psychological and social factors (e.g., depression, social isolation) affecting use of and response to drugs may make the elderly more prone to medication errors than are younger patients (Klein, German & Levine 1981).

Although adverse drug reactions may occur with a single drug, they may also occur as a result of drug-drug interactions. Elderly patients are at greater risk for drug-drug interactions because they often have more than one chronic condition and thus take multiple drugs. They also may be using prescription and nonprescription drugs simultaneously. The drugs that are most likely to produce clinically significant drug-drug interactions include anticoagulants, cardiac drugs (e.g., digoxin), anticonvulsants (especially phenytoin), histamine antagonists (e.g., cimetidine), nonsteroidal antiinflammatory drugs, and alcohol.

The clinical characteristics of drug-drug interactions have been described by Hansten (1986) and may be summarized as follows:

□ Drug-drug reactions exhibit high interpatient variability.

□ They are difficult to detect.

□ They seldom represent a contraindication to continued use but may require adjustments in the dosage or dosage timing.

□ Most such interactions are dose-related.

□ The adverse effects are seldom immediate.

□ They may be caused because individual drugs within a drug class may not interact in a homogeneous manner with other drugs.

Many drug-drug interactions are predictable, based on the alterations in pharmacokinetics and pharmacodynamics caused by aging (Lamy 1986). Adverse drug reactions are more likely to occur in the elderly not only because of the elderly's altered response to drugs but also because of reduction in the efficiency of the body's homeostatic mechanisms. For example, impaired baroreceptor function makes the elderly more liable to drug-induced postural hypotension, while the reduced capacity of temperature-regulating mechanisms may result in drug-induced hypothermia. Other areas of homeostatic function may also be impaired with aging and create a greater likelihood of adverse drug reactions.

No satisfactory method has yet been developed for assembling meaningful national or international statistics on adverse drug reactions, and national health statistics in the United States do not reflect the magnitude of the problem of drug-induced illnesses. The limitations of current data cause some clinicians to doubt that adverse drug reactions among the elderly present a significant problem (Karsh 1980; Klein, German & Levine 1981). However, such reactions have long been considered a major medical problem by many clinicians and investigators (Moser 1964; Melmon 1974; Silverman & Lee 1974; Cluff 1980). We believe that the evidence is sufficient to warrant the attention of all clinicians who have elderly patients. We also believe that there is a need to establish and maintain a substantial base of information on patterns of drug use and adverse drug reactions among the elderly in order to deal with the problem more effectively.

The best information on adverse drug reactions has been gathered by the Boston Collaborative Drug Surveillance Program (BCDSP). An adverse drug reaction developed in about 30 percent of the 45,000 hospital inpatients who had been admitted to the medical wards in the fifty hospitals monitored by the BCDSP (Jick et al. 1970; R. R.

Miller 1973; Jick 1974, 1986). For each course of therapy (the patients received, on average, nine drugs each during hospitalization), the chances of an adverse drug reaction were 5 percent. The most frequently observed reactions were nausea, drowsiness, diarrhea, vomiting, rash, arrhythmia, itching, injection site complication, hyperkalemia, and drug fever (Jick 1986).

Although most of the adverse drug reactions were transient and of minor importance, about 3 percent of the patients monitored by the BCDSP had serious, life-threatening reactions. The frequency per course of drug treatment was 0.4 percent (R. R. Miller 1973). The most common life-threatening adverse drug reactions were arrhythmia, bone marrow depression, central nervous system depression, hemorrhage, renal failure, hyperkalemia, hypotension, and fluid and electrolyte disturbances (Jick 1986).

Estimates indicate that adverse drug reactions are the direct cause of from 1 to 3 percent of all medical admissions to hospitals in the United States (R. R. Miller 1973). Based on the assumption that 75 million adults take, on average, two drugs regularly and that 300,000 hospitalizations each year result from adverse drug reactions, Jick estimated that hospitalization results from 1 out of every 500 regular drug treatments.

Epidemiological evidence indicates that the elderly are at particular risk for adverse drug reactions. In a three-year study of hospital admissions in a large university teaching hospital, adverse drug reactions were responsible for 3 percent of all admissions. The hospital admission rate due to drug-induced illness among elderly patients was fifteen times that in the younger age group (Caranasos, Stewart & Cluff 1974).

Furthermore, the elderly are at least twice as likely as are younger patients to suffer an adverse drug reaction while already in the hospital. In a study of 700 hospitalized patients, drug-induced illness was found in 25 percent of patients older than 80 years of age, as compared with 12 percent of patients 21 to 50 years of age (Seidl et al. 1966). In another study of 815 hospitalized patients, researchers found a prevalence rate of 36 percent for iatrogenic illnesses, almost half of which were caused by drugs. Of these drug complications, 6 to 9 percent were categorized as "major" or "severe." Increased length of stay was related to the adverse drug reaction rate, and, significantly, patients suffering such reactions were likely to be elderly (Steel et al. 1981).

Drugs Causing Adverse Drug Reactions

Although a wide variety of drugs may cause adverse reactions, there are four classes of drugs that must be used with special caution in the elderly: (1) antihypertensives, (2) antiparkinson drugs, (3) psychotropics, and (4) cardiac glycosides—for example, digoxin (Williamson & Chopin 1980). Antibiotics, because of their widespread overuse, are also likely to present problems in the elderly (Lamy 1984). It is difficult to detect adverse drug reactions in the elderly because many common symptoms associated with chronic illness and functional disability in old age can be drug-induced (Table 1.1).

A clear relation of age to adverse effects has been demonstrated for two tranquilizers—chlordiazepoxide and diazepam (Boston Collab-

TABLE 1.1

Drugs Regularly Detected as Causing Adverse Reactions in the Elderly

CONFUSIONAL STATES
hypnotics, tranquilizers, antidepressants, antipsychotics, anticholinergics (centrally acting), nonsteroidal antiinflammatory drugs, levodopa, bromocriptine, antidiabetics (hypoglycemia), corticosteroids, digitalis glycosides, phenytoin, cimetidine

DEPRESSION
methyldopa, reserpine, beta-blockers, tranquilizers, levodopa, corticosteroids

FALLS
hypnotics, tranquilizers, antidepressants, antipsychotics, antihistamines, carbamazepine, phenytoin, phenobarbital, all drugs liable to produce postural hypotension, glyceryl trinitrate

POSTURAL HYPOTENSION
all antihypertensives, diuretics, antianginal drugs, beta-blockers, hypnotics, tranquilizers, antidepressants, antipsychotics, antihistamines, levodopa, bromocriptine

CONSTIPATION
dextropropoxyphene, narcotic analgesics, diuretics, anticholinergics, disopyramide, verapamil, nifedipine, antidepressants, antipsychotics

URINARY INCONTINENCE
diuretics, hypnotics, tranquilizers, antipsychotics, prazosin, labetalol, all drugs liable to produce fecal impaction, beta-blockers

PARKINSONISM
antipsychotics, drugs for vertigo, methyldopa, reserpine, metoclopramide

SOURCE: World Health Organization 1985: 25.

orative Drug Surveillance Program 1973). This relation between age and adverse effects also exists for the sleeping pill flurazepam (Greenblatt, Allen & Shader 1977) and for the anticoagulant heparin (Jick et al. 1968). Drug-induced admissions to the hospital have also been found among the elderly who use the anticoagulant warfarin, the cardiac drug digoxin, the diuretics furosemide and hydrochlorothiazide, the anticancer drug vincristine, the corticosteroid prednisone, and aspirin. Serious adverse reactions may occur when a drug is used frequently (e.g., hydrochlorthiazide and the nonsteroidal antiinflammatory drugs, including aspirin), when the balance between a toxic and a therapeutic dose is narrow (e.g., digoxin), or when the drug is toxic even at doses required to produce clinical benefits (e.g., many anticancer drugs). Other drugs causing severe or unusual side effects, such as barbiturates and the antiinflammatory drug phenylbutazone, should also be avoided (World Health Organization 1985).

In nursing homes, adverse drug reactions are related primarily to the widespread use of psychotropic drugs and the use of multiple drugs simultaneously. Several studies have shown increased toxicity from psychotropic drugs among the elderly (Boston Collaborative Drug Surveillance Program 1973; Davies 1971; Greenblatt, Allen & Shader 1977). These drugs are used in the majority of nursing home patients. Elderly patients in nursing homes are also at risk because they are prescribed multiple drugs. For example, of the 512 nursing home patients surveyed by Blaschke and his colleagues, the average number of drugs received per patient was six, with 20 percent of the patients receiving potentially interacting combinations (Blaschke et al. 1981). The more drugs prescribed per patient, the greater is the likelihood of an interacting combination resulting in an adverse drug reaction.

Alcohol and Drugs

Alcohol intake by the elderly may complicate the use of both prescription and nonprescription drugs (Lamy 1986). Several problems may arise: the synergistic effect of alcohol and drugs, increased adverse drug reactions due to drug-alcohol interaction, and the well-documented effect of alcohol on drug metabolism (Salerno 1980).

Synergistic effects with alcohol are found most commonly with depressant drugs, such as sedatives, tranquilizers, narcotic analgesics, antihistamines, and muscle relaxants. The synergistic effects are perhaps best illustrated by the combined effects of alcohol and phenobarbital. In humans, lethal serum ethyl alcohol levels range from 500 mg/ 100 ml to 800 mg/100 ml, and lethal phenobarbital levels normally range from 10 to 30 mg/100 ml. When alcohol and phenobarbital are consumed in combination, the fatal serum ethyl alcohol level may be as low as 100 mg/ml and the fatal phenobarbital level as low as .5 mg/100 ml (Seixas 1975).

Adverse drug reactions may also occur when alcohol is used with aspirin, a drug commonly used to treat arthritis symptoms. Alcohol used in combination with aspirin may precipitate gastrointestinal bleeding by enhancing the irritant effect of aspirin on gastric or duodenal mucosa. Alcohol may also increase the risk of bleeding associated with warfarin. Patients who are taking aspirin or other salicylates and patients for whom warfarin has been prescribed should not use alcohol.

In addition, alcohol, because of its vasodilation effect, may enhance the absorption of nitroglycerine or other nitrates. Alcohol may also result in hypotension in patients using nitrates for the treatment of angina pectoris. Because elderly patients with angina pectoris may use nitrates frequently and/or inconsistently, they should be told of the problems associated with alcohol consumption.

Physicians and pharmacists have limited control over their patients' drinking or use of such nonprescription medicines as aspirin. They should, however, be aware of the risks and advise patients accordingly. Pharmacists, in particular, are in a position to advise patients about the selection of nonprescription drugs (e.g., acetaminophen instead of aspirin) that may be used safely with alcohol.

Nutritional Status of the Elderly and Their Response to Drugs

The nutritional status of elderly people is adversely affected by a variety of factors, including poverty, social isolation, lack of adequate exercise, and biological changes associated with aging. The reduced sensitivity of the taste buds and olfactory receptor cells decreases the flavor of food, making it less appealing, and loss of teeth or poorly fitting dentures encourages a reliance on soft processed foods. Chronic disease may alter nutritional requirements. Moreover, there may be a long history of poor eating habits continuing into old age.

Drugs are also capable of altering nutrient intake or utilization. Among the classes of drugs affecting nutrition are antacids, antidepressants, anorexiants, antimicrobials, laxatives, corticosteroids, cytotoxic agents, diuretics, anticonvulsants, hypocholesteremic agents, and antipsychotics (Yosselson 1976). Drugs may affect nutrition in four ways: (1) impaired absorption of nutrients when used for prolonged periods of time, (2) impaired utilization of nutrients, (3) reactions with pharmacologically active ingredients in foods, and (4) altered food intake. However, it is important to note that if the elderly person is given proper counseling and if appropriate vitamins or other nutritional supplements are used, drugs may be taken with little nutritional risk (Javert & Macri 1941; Christakis & Miridjanian 1958).

Impaired Absorption of Nutrients

Drugs that lower blood cholesterol (e.g., Neomycin, clofibrate, and cholestyramine) have been associated with a variety of malabsorption problems including diminished vitamin B-12 and iron absorption (Krondl 1970). Mineral oil, when used regularly as a laxative, may decrease the absorption of vitamins A, D, E, and K (Javert & Macri 1941; Christakis & Miridjanian 1958). Excessive use of antacids may reduce thiamine absorption. Colchicine, used in the treatment of gout, may impair vitamin B-12 absorption (Cooper 1976).

Impaired Utilization of Nutrients

The utilization of nutrients after absorption may be adversely affected by a number of drugs. Phenytoin and phenobarbital, both used to treat patients with epilepsy, have been found to impair folic acid utilization (Reilly 1970). Pyridoxine utilization is affected by isoniazid, used to treat patients with tuberculosis. Without pyridoxine replacement, neurological symptoms may develop in patients receiving long-term treatment. Vitamin D is also affected by phenytoin. Thiamine levels may be reduced in patients receiving cardiac glycosides chronically. Although many other drug-nutrient interactions are known to occur and can cause similar problems, there seems to be minimal danger of vitamin deficiency diseases, for these are rarely seen in connection with prescription drugs.

Reactions with Pharmacologically Active
Substances in Food

Some foods containing a pharmacologically active substance, if consumed along with certain drugs, may produce an unexpected effect. A clinically important example of this type of interaction, documented in large numbers of cases, is the hypertensive reaction caused by patients who eat foods rich in tyramines (e.g., red wine, aged cheeses, chicken livers) while taking monoamine oxidase (MAO) inhibitors (e.g., tranylcypromine and phenelzine) for the treatment of depression. Hypertensive symptoms range from headaches and nosebleeds to death from cerebrovascular accidents. Although these drugs were not commonly used to treat elderly depressed patients in the past, there is now renewed interest in their use in the treatment of depression. Thus, it is very important that elderly patients receiving MAO inhibitors be counseled regarding their diets.

Other foods involved in drug-food interactions include natural licorice, which produces sodium retention; green, leafy vegetables, which, when consumed in large amounts, may alter the response to anticoagulant therapy; and caffeine-containing foods (e.g., coffee, tea, cola drinks), which may interact with numerous drugs by enhancing their stimulant effect. For example, the combination of the bronchodilator theophyllin and coffee may cause insomnia, nervousness, or palpitations in an individual who would not be affected by either substance taken alone.

The Effect of Drugs on Food Intake

Food intake may be reduced by those drugs that produce gastric irritation or nausea. Loss of appetite and/or nausea is an early sign of digoxin toxicity. Drugs that affect the sense of smell or taste (e.g., d-penicillamine, penicillin tablets, or sympathomimetic nasal sprays and drops) also have an adverse effect on food intake (Pierpaoli et al. 1976).

The Aging Body and Drugs—Priorities for Research

Psychological and social changes accompanying aging may be as important as biological changes in determining an elderly person's response to drugs. Yet these factors have received scant attention by clinicians or investigators. Clinical, psychological, and sociological studies are needed to identify problems and to develop improved methods of drug management.

Similarly, clinical investigators have not paid enough attention to the interrelationships among the biological, psychological, and social changes brought about by age. We must learn more of these dynamics to determine how they affect the elderly's responses to drugs and how they affect drug prescribing, dispensing, and administration.

Other areas requiring study relate to differences in body composition (e.g., the proportion of fat) with respect to age and sex, and changes in drug metabolism in the liver with aging. Although it is clear that the liver's capacity to metabolize and clear drugs is altered with increasing age, it is difficult to predict the clinical significance of these changes. In addition, we need studies on the clinical effects of the use of specific drugs with alcohol, nicotine, and caffeine, because the latter are used widely and affect reactions to prescribed drugs.

Drug testing guidelines related to the elderly are currently under review by the FDA. The proposed guidelines require that drugs be tested among the elderly before the FDA approves them for marketing (see Chapter 6). Should the proposed guidelines be approved, the pharmaceutical industry and clinical investigators in medical schools, pharmacy schools, and other academic or health care institutions will doubtless become more involved in expanded drug testing of the elderly. Such activity can only enhance our knowledge of the aging body's response to drugs—a much needed development.

CHAPTER TWO

Patterns of Geriatric Drug Use
and Factors Affecting Use

Introduction

I n this chapter we describe patterns of prescription and non-prescription drug use among the population in general and among the elderly in particular. We analyze drug use in geriatric populations and factors affecting use, discuss some of the issues associated with widespread use, and assess the status of current research. The focus of this chapter is on geriatric drug use in ambulatory care settings—settings outside hospitals and nursing homes. Issues related to geriatric drug misuse, particularly prevalent in hospitals and nursing homes, are considered in the next chapter.

The consumption of prescription and nonprescription drugs is almost universal. The two most important factors affecting the widespread use of drugs are the growing number of elderly persons and their burden of disease, discomfort, and disability. Another factor affecting drug use is the prevalence of self-care, which is widespread among the entire population (Alonzo 1979; Verbrugge & Ascione 1987). Of every 100 adults, 75 experience at least one episode of ill health or injury each month. Only 25 consult a physician about their symptoms (White, Williams & Greenberg 1961). The vast majority of adults who do not seek professional medical consultation for illness or injury use nonprescription drugs.

The Use of Nonprescription Drugs

The use of nonprescription drugs constitutes an important component of self-care: 70 percent of all illnesses are treated with nonprescription drugs (Knapp & Knapp 1972). Nonprescription drugs tend to be used primarily for fever, fatigue, headache and other aches, sore throat, and digestive problems (e.g., indigestion, constipation). This is hardly surprising in view of the extent of media advertising for analgesics, cold remedies, antacids, and laxatives.

The total cost of nonprescription drugs bought by consumers is about one-half that of drugs prescribed by physicians—a statistic that reflects the lower price of nonprescription drugs. In 1984 about 56 percent of the $26 billion spent for drugs and drug sundries in noninstitutional settings in the United States was spent for prescription drugs, and 29 percent for nonprescription drugs. The remaining 15 percent was spent for a variety of medical sundries (D. Waldo, Health Care Financing Administration, letter of Feb. 19, 1986).

Nonprescription Drugs and the Elderly

Drug purchasing increases with age. However, purchasing of nonprescription drugs reportedly peaks at age 65 years and begins to taper off, whereas purchasing of prescription drugs continues to increase (Lamy 1979; May et al. 1982; Bush & Rabin 1976; Bush & Osterweis 1978). This pattern may result from the substitution of prescription for nonprescription drugs by the elderly who are chronically ill. Another explanation may be the attitude of the elderly: a 1972 FDA survey indicated that older consumers believe prescription medicines to be safer than nonprescription medicines (Knapp 1974).

Although the ratio of prescription to nonprescription drug use may change with age, the majority of elderly persons still use nonprescription drugs. One survey showed that two-thirds of the elderly use nonprescription drugs; oral analgesics made up over half of these drugs, and cough-and-cold preparations about 13 percent. Of the subjects surveyed, less than 10 percent relied on nonprescription drugs to perform daily activities, but 40 percent claimed such reliance on prescription drugs (Guttmann 1977). From this, we may conclude that the nonprescription drugs were not essential and were, perhaps, even unnecessary. Almost half of the elderly subjects in another study took vitamins (Rose et al. 1976). Yet another study of drug use in an ambulatory geriatric population found that 70 percent of the women and 58 percent of the men were taking at least one nonprescription medication. Of the most commonly used nonprescription drugs, the top five were aspirin, multiple vitamins, vitamin E, multiple vitamins with minerals, and vitamin C. The investigators, in questioning whether these vitamin and mineral supplements are needed by the elderly, asserted that proper nutrition might be a more worthwhile investment than large expenditures on vitamin and mineral supplements (May et al. 1982).

Nonprescription drug use in itself does not appear to be dangerous (Blum & Kreitman 1981). However, the risk of adverse effects is increased for those patients who combine prescription and nonprescription drugs and for those who use several nonprescription drugs simultaneously.

Factors Affecting the Use of Nonprescription Drugs

Factors that influence the use of nonprescription drugs differ from those that affect the use of prescribed medicines. Nonprescription drug use is usually patient-initiated, although physicians and pharmacists may sometimes recommend nonprescription drugs. Family, self-care, and self-help groups strongly influence decisions about drug use (Levin & Idler 1981).

Attempts to explain the use of nonprescription drugs by correlating use to variables such as socioeconomic status have not proved successful. Few such variables show a consistent correlation. For example, although persons with higher incomes may purchase more drugs than do those with lower incomes, actual use of nonprescription drugs does not seem to be tied to income (Svarstad 1983). Some researchers have found that nonprescription drugs are used least frequently by people of high socioeconomic status (Koos 1954); some have found the opposite to be true (Salber et al. 1979); and some have found no difference (Knapp & Knapp 1972). A few studies have found that the higher the level of education, the greater is the use of nonprescription drugs (Jefferys, Brotherston & Cartwright 1960; Quah 1977), but no consistent results have been reported with respect to race (Bush & Rabin 1976; Salber et al. 1979) or marital status (Rabin 1972; Murray 1973).

Even the expected relationship between self-reported health status and self-medication has not been firmly established. While most studies suggest that sick people use more nonprescription drugs than do healthy people (Bush & Rabin 1976; Dunnell & Cartwright 1972), other studies have found that healthy people take more nonprescription drugs than do sick people (Rabin & Bush 1974; Wadsworth, Butterfield & Blaney 1971). Although it is difficult to know the reason for these inconsistent findings, it is important to note that in absolute terms, many nonprescription drug users report themselves as healthy (Dunnell & Cartwright 1972; Bush & Rabin 1976).

Theoretical models, such as the behavioral and stress models, have been proposed to explain nonprescription drug use. The behavioral model, developed by Andersen (1968) and adapted by Bush and Osterweis (1978), assumes that three distinct sets of factors influence nonprescription drug use: predisposing factors (e.g., age and sex); enabling factors (e.g., access to private or public health insurance coverage); and need factors (e.g., morbidity). The model is of limited usefulness because it explains very little of the total variation in nonprescription drug use (Svarstad 1983).

According to the stress hypothesis, life stress and psychological distress are precursors to nonprescription drug use. Life stress involves events that can be experienced as difficult (e.g., loss of job or spouse). These difficult events, which are external to the individual, can cause psychological distress. Psychological distress involves people's symptomatic and somatic reactions to life stress (e.g., anxiety, depression, insomnia). In general, studies exploring the stress hypothesis have proved to be of limited value in explaining the use of nonprescription drugs (Svarstad 1983). The most serious difficulty is the failure of researchers to control for variables such as health status. In addition, investigators often rely on specialized populations and nonstandardized or biased procedures for evaluating patients' psychological well-being. Then, too, because few, if any, of the studies make a clear distinction between life stress and psychological distress, the research leaves unanswered questions about the impact of these variables on nonprescription drug use. Nor do the studies adequately examine the relationship between stress and variation in drug use (e.g., type of drug used, amount of use, duration of use, etc.).

To overcome these problems, Svarstad (1983) selected a Wisconsin community in which she conducted an epidemiological study of the relationship between life stress, psychological stress, and the use of nonprescription drugs. Results revealed that both types of stress are significantly related to nonprescription drug use, even when socioeconomic status, attitudes, access to medical care, and health status were controlled. The study goes beyond previous work by demonstrating that certain forms of distress are strongly predictive of the use of particular classes of nonprescription drugs. For example, analgesic users tend to be anxious and depressed, whereas vitamin users are likely to suffer from insomnia and fatigue. These findings suggest that people do not use nonprescription drugs in an indiscriminate fashion but rather select a drug to "fit" their symptoms and their perceptions of how their problems might be relieved.

The Use of Prescription Drugs

Use of prescription drugs is widespread among the general population. Drugs are prescribed in over 60 percent of all visits to office-based physicians (Koch 1982). During a typical hospital stay, a patient takes about nine prescription drugs (Lee 1981a; Jick 1986). However, prescription drug use is even more widespread among the elderly. In nursing homes, for example, over 95 percent of the patients receive prescription drugs (Cooper 1981).

From the mid-1940s until the mid-1970s, the use of prescription drugs rose steadily in the United States. The number of prescriptions dispensed by community pharmacies rose from approximately 363 million in 1950 to 634 million in 1960, to 1.28 billion in 1970, and to a peak of 1.52 billion in 1973. The number of prescriptions declined gradually after the mid-1970s to 1.38 billion in 1979 (*Pharmacy Times* 1980). This decline was only temporary, for the number of prescriptions increased again in 1980 and rose to 1.55 billion in 1985 (*Pharmacy Times* 1986).

Using estimates of overall drug use from 1972 through 1981, analysts from the Food and Drug Administration found that the downward trend in total number of prescriptions in the mid-1970s appears to have been related to a steady rise in prescription size—the number of tablets, capsules, or other units included in the prescription (Baum et al. 1984). Drug industry statistics indicate that prescription size has, in fact, risen steadily since 1960 and that the average 1981 prescription contained 27 percent more units (e.g., tablets or capsules) than the average 1971 prescription. If increasing prescription size is considered, the apparent decline in prescription drug use from 1973 through 1979 occurred only from 1977 to 1979 and was followed by an increase in 1980 and 1981 (Baum et al. 1984).

Factors Influencing Drug Prescribing and Use

What factors contribute to the increasing use of prescription drugs? Certainly the growth in the number of elderly persons and their burden of chronic illness. A primary-care physician is likely to have 10,000 patient visits in a year. Of these, 10 to 15 percent involve major acute illnesses, 35 to 45 percent involve minor acute conditions, and 40 percent involve chronic conditions. Patients with chronic conditions are more likely to require prescription drugs than are those with self-limited acute illnesses, and the elderly, of course, are more likely to have chronic conditions.

Another important factor contributing to use of prescription drugs has been the development during the past 65 years of a broad spectrum of safe and effective drugs from which physicians can choose. Drug companies also play a critical role in drug use by influencing physician prescribing. They communicate with physicians in two key ways: through professional sales representatives (often called detail persons), who call on physicians, and through advertising in professional journals. Communication also takes place through direct mailings, medical conventions, industry-sponsored lectures and seminars, as well as radio, television, and magazine advertising.

The nature of the physician-patient relationship and the expectations each brings to the encounter also influence decisions about drug use. Patients bring complaints to physicians and expect relief. Patients who are regular users of long-term, repeat prescriptions want to feel that their visit to the physician is worthwhile, so physicians oblige with a prescription. The prescription is a tangible act that acknowledges the patient's need. It reflects the physician's concern for the patient, and it allows the office visit to end in a manner recognized as legitimate by both patient and physician (Mueller 1972).

For many physicians and patients, prescribing legitimizes a patient's complaints as medical. In the absence of a prescription, the patient's problem might be perceived as a personal or social matter outside the domain of medicine and not justifying the visit to the physician. For the aged, many of whom lead lives of social isolation, the request or need for a prescription provides an excuse for human contact. It can open the door to discussion of personal, even intimate, matters with the physician. The prescription also can become a reaffirmation of care in a long-term illness without cure. It avoids the conclusion that "nothing can be done" or that the problem is "psychological"—attitudes that many elderly regard as stigmatizing. Thus, for some patients who are regular users of long-term repeat prescriptions, drugs eliminate the need for psychotherapy, while permitting continuing human contact with a physician (Pellegrino 1976).

Factors such as income, education, marital status, family size, and geographic setting (urban, rural, etc.) have been related to the number of drugs used but do not show consistent correlations (U.S. Department of Health, Education, and Welfare 1969; Rabin 1972; Kalimo 1969; Dunnell & Cartwright 1972; Stolley et al. 1972; U.S.

Department of Health, Education, and Welfare 1974; Bush & Rabin 1976; Bush & Osterweis 1978). Age and gender, however, are closely associated with physicians' drug prescribing and patients' drug use (Johnson & Azevedo 1979; Lech, Friedman & Ury 1975). In the next sections we review studies that have been conducted among different patient populations and in varied health care settings to determine the influence of age and gender on prescription drug use.

Age as a Factor in Drug Use: Number of Drugs Prescribed

Data consistently indicate that the elderly use more drugs than do younger people. Patients aged 65 years and older, although they constitute only about 11 percent of the population, received 31 percent of all prescriptions in 1981 (Baum et al. 1984). The relationship between age and drug use was apparent in the results of a national survey conducted by the National Center for Health Services Research. Results revealed that of those people receiving prescriptions from a physician, the average number of prescriptions in 1977 was 7.5 per person, but 14.2 prescriptions per elderly person (Kasper 1982).

The relationship between age and drug use has to do with an inescapable fact of life for people over 65: 80 percent of the elderly have one or more chronic illnesses, and close to half of those with chronic illnesses are limited in their daily activities. This latter group is particularly vulnerable: the 46 percent of the elderly limited in their activities accounted for 63 percent of physician visits, 71 percent of hospitalizations, and 82 percent of all the days spent in bed by the elderly because of ill health (Rice & Estes 1984). The elderly restricted in activity because of chronic illness are far more likely to need prescription drugs than are the healthy elderly or younger groups.

Drugs Prescribed Most Often

A survey done by the National Center for Health Statistics showed that of the 2,600 different drugs and drug categories prescribed by physicians in 1980, 8 percent, or 200 drugs and drug categories, accounted for nearly two-thirds of all drug use (Koch 1982). The three categories from which most drugs were prescribed were central nervous system drugs (e.g., tranquilizers), accounting for 16.3 percent of drug use; antiinfective agents (basically antibiotics), accounting for 15.4 percent of use; and cardiovascular drugs (such as cardiac drugs and antihypertensive drugs), accounting for 9.5 percent. A different picture emerged, however, when drug use was examined according to age and gender: cardiovascular drugs and diuretics were the major therapeutic categories in male and female groups aged 65 and over (see Table 2.1).

Additional data on drug use by the elderly are presented in Table 2.2, which provides a list of drug categories most frequently prescribed for patients in different age groups (Baum, Kennedy & Forbes 1985). These data represent only outpatient prescription drug use and do not include prescriptions dispensed from outlets other than retail pharmacies. The most commonly prescribed drugs for persons aged 65 to 74 are systemic antiarthritics, followed by cardiovascular drugs, including beta-blockers, thiazide, and related diuretics. Digitalis preparations are the drugs most commonly prescribed for persons 75 years of age and older. Drugs used in cardiovascular therapy (e.g., antihypertensives, antiarrhythmics, antianginals) ranked high for both the age groups over 64 because of the prevalence of hypertension and heart disease among the elderly and the increased availability of drugs to treat these conditions.

Digitalis and "other oral diuretics" (mainly furosemide) are the only categories in Table 2.2 that show a consistent increase in use with age. The rankings for thiazide diuretics, potassium-sparing diuretics, and "other antihypertensives" are remarkably similar across the four older age groups, and nitrite or nitrate coronary vasodilators have identical rankings for the three age groups 55 years and older. The two oldest age groups have very similar rankings. Exceptions are beta-blockers, insulin, and antidepressants, which drop in rankings in the oldest age group, and digitalis and "other oral diuretics," which rise in rankings in the oldest age group.

Use of Psychotropic Drugs

The elderly living outside institutions are assumed to be heavy users of psychotropic drugs, but data do not support this view. Actually, the majority of elderly do not use these drugs (Stephens, Haney & Underwood 1982). Although psychotropic drug use is greater among middle-aged and older persons than among those less than 50 years of age, the precise relation of age to use differs among drug classes (Mellinger & Balter 1981). Use of antianxiety agents (minor tranquilizers) is most common among persons 50 to 64 years of age

TABLE 2.1

Number of Drug Mentions and Drug Mention Rate Per 1,000 Visits for the 10 Drugs Most Frequently Ordered or Provided to Patients 65 and Over, United States, 1980

Rank	Entry name and generic name (in parentheses) of drug	No. of mentions (000)	Drug mention rate per 1,000 visits	Rank	Entry name and generic name (in parentheses) of drug	No. of mentions (000)	Drug mention rate per 1,000 visits
	Female patients 65 years and older				*Male patients 65 years and older*		
1	Lanoxin (digoxin)	3,089	50.8	1	Lasix (furosemide)	2,247	56.6
2	Lasix (furosemide)	2,931	48.2	2	Lanoxin (digoxin)	2,078	52.3
3	Dyazide (triamterene)	2,613	43.0	3	Inderal (propranolol)	1,609	40.5
4	Inderal (propranolol)	2,576	42.4	4	Digoxin	1,512	38.1
5	Aldomet (methyldopa)	2,067	34.0	5	Isordil (isosorbide)	1,143	28.8
6	Vitamin B-12 [a]	1,987	32.7	6	Dyazide (triamterene)	956	24.1
7	Digoxin	1,793	29.5	7	Aspirin [b]	765	19.3
8	Motrin (ibuprofen)	1,467	24.1	8	Hydrochlorothiazide	761	19.2
9	Insulin	1,382	22.7	9	Hydrodiuril (hydrochlorothiazide)	742	18.7
10	Hydrochlorothiazide	1,340	22.0	10	Prednisone	715	18.0

SOURCE: National Center for Health Statistics & Bloom (1982): 7.

NOTE: "Drug mention rate" is the average number of drugs ordered or provided per office visit.

[a] Vitamin B-12 is often prescribed for the treatment of pernicious anemia.

[b] Although vitamins and aspirin are considered nonprescription drugs, they can be prescribed by physicians for treatment of certain conditions and to ensure that the patient is taking a certain dosage, is on a certain schedule, etc.

TABLE 2.2

Drug Groups Ranked by Frequency of Use in Age Groups

Drug groups (USC category)	Frequency of use in age group				
	Under 45	45–54	55–64	65–74	75+
Systemic antiarthritics	8	1	2	1	2
Beta-blockers	20	2	1	2	6
Thiazide and related diuretics	28	3	3	3	4
Digitalis preparations	99	34	9	4	1
Potassium-sparing diuretics	49	5	4	5	5
Other oral diuretics (e.g., furosemide)	78	18	8	6	3
Other antihypertensives (e.g., methyldopa)	73	8	5	8	8
Nitrate/nitrite coronary vasodilators	a	16	7	7	7
Benzodiazepine tranquilizers	14	4	6	10	12
Diabetes therapy, oral	100	17	11	9	9
Codeine and combinations, oral analgesics	10	6	9	15	6
Plain corticoids, oral	15	12	13	14	15
Xanthine bronchodilators	18	23	14	11	13
Diabetes therapy, insulin	56	19	12	12	21
Tricyclic and related antidepressants	17	7	15	20	27

SOURCE: *National Disease and Therapeutic Index*, IMS America, Ltd. 1982 (as cited in Baum, Kennedy & Forbes 1985: 65). The National Disease and Therapeutic Index (NDTI) is based on a panel of approximately 2,000 private office-based physicians who report on every contact they have with a patient during a specified two-day period.
a Not in top 100.

and seems to decline slightly beyond that age. Use of antipsychotics (major tranquilizers) is not clearly or consistently related to age (Koch 1983). Use of hypnotics (sleeping pills), however, is most common among 65- to 79-year-olds.

Although psychotropic drug use among the elderly living outside institutions does not appear to be a significant public health problem, evidence suggests that once a person in this age group begins to use a psychotropic drug, there is a reasonable chance of "misuse"—that is, of long-term continuous use. Traditionally, psychotropic drugs are not intended for long-term use because of the risk of physical dependence or reduced efficacy of the drug.

To determine who uses psychotropic drugs on a long-term basis, Mellinger and his colleagues analyzed data derived from their 1979 national survey of noninstitutionalized adults (Mellinger & Balter 1981). Analysis of users of antianxiety drugs revealed that long-term use (defined as regular daily use for a year or longer) was relatively rare, occurring among 15 percent of all such users. This represents only 1.6 percent of all surveyed adults between the ages of 18 and 79 years (Mellinger, Balter & Uhlenhuth 1984). Similarly, the researchers found that a minority of users of sedative-hypnotics reported daily use of these medications for periods of time longer than present clinical standards justify. (Most patients should not use sedative-hypnotics except for short-term treatment, usually not exceeding two weeks.) Since several studies indicate that the elderly are major users of sleeping pills (Basen 1977; Koch 1983), it is probable that many of the people in the Mellinger survey who used sleeping pills for excessively long periods of time were elderly.

In their analysis of users of antianxiety drugs, Mellinger and his colleagues noted a striking difference between long-term users and others: the long-term user was older. Of the long-term users, 71 percent were 50 years of age and older, compared with 48 percent of other users and 34 percent of nonusers. A third of the long-term users were 65 years of age or older.

The long-term user of antianxiety drugs was characterized as having high levels of emotional distress and chronic somatic health problems. Long-term users were somewhat more likely to be males than were short-term and occasional users. Many of these patients were sufficiently distressed to seek other sources of help—other psychotropic medications or mental health professionals. Most long-term users were monitored by their physicians at intervals not longer than four months—the time at which physicians are urged to reevaluate the need to continue this kind of medication (Mellinger, Balter & Uhlenhuth 1984).

The major physical health problems of long-term antianxiety drug users were likely to be chronic. Almost half reported a major health problem in one of two categories of chronic illness: cardiovascular disease and arthritis. The prevalence of these illnesses was about 50 percent higher among long-term users than among occasional users and about 2.5 times that found among nonusers. The Mellinger group believes that this finding supports their contention that the most widely used psychotropic drugs are frequently prescribed in cases in which physicians are treating a physical condition that may also be connected to emotional distress. In short, these data imply that use of antianxiety agents is strongly associated with real health problems that are physical, as well as emotional, in nature.

One hypothesis concerning patterns of drug use by the elderly is the layering effect model (Zawadski, Glazer & Lurie 1978). According to this model, there is a baseline level of drug use for the general population—antacids, antibiotics, analgesics, and vitamins. For the noninstitutionalized, chronically ill elderly another layer is added—antihypertensives, diuretics, antidiabetics, and other medicines for treatment of chronic diseases. For the institutionalized elderly and a small percentage of ambulatory patients with chronic medical and psychosocial problems, yet another layer is observed—psychotropic drugs, including major tranquilizers and sedatives.

Although the layering effect model describes drug use by the elderly, it does not explain why tranquilizers are prescribed for elderly patients with chronic disease. Nor does it examine whether chronic illnesses are necessarily compatible with psychotropic drug treatment. Further, although patients using these medications report regular consultations with their physicians, there is no guarantee that physicians adequately monitor drug use during office visits. Finally, the model does not predict the conditions under which persons using these medications experience adverse reactions.

Gender as a Factor in Drug Use

Studies have long reported higher levels of drug use in females than in males of all ages over 14 years (Whittington et al. 1982; Rabin & Bush 1975; Rowe 1973; Prentice 1979). This finding is consistent even after symptomatology and frequency of physician consultations have been taken into account. A study comparing older females' use of prescribed medication with that of males found that women took significantly more drugs than did men. Unable to explain the gender-based difference in drug use, the authors suggested that further research be done on social factors and on the behavior of health professionals in their treatment of older men and women (Whittington et al. 1982).

Data published by the National Center for Health Statistics' National Ambulatory Medical Care Survey demonstrate greater psychotropic drug use by women than by men. This national survey of office-based ambulatory care found that general use of psychotropics is equivalent for females and males who are 45 years of age or younger. For persons 45 or older, however, use differs dramatically. In the group aged 45 to 64 years, female use is roughly one-third higher than is male use, and in the group 65 years and over, female use exceeds male use by almost 60 percent. This latter finding also holds true for those 75 years of age and older (Koch & Smith 1985). These findings correlate positively with the evidence that emotional disorders and essential hypertension—conditions that command the highest rate of psychotropic drug use—were more common among older female patients than among males (Koch 1983). The use of these drugs among women, in contrast to that among men, appears to be primarily on a short-term basis.

Greater psychotropic drug use by women is not confined to the community setting. A study of elderly persons in a long-term care facility found that females were more likely than males to receive major tranquilizers and to be defined as anxious. The author concluded that sex roles and the expectations of health personnel regarding the behavior of men and women are significant factors affecting prescribing and dispensing of tranquilizers in long-term care facilities (Milleren 1977).

Gender and Drug Use: Some Unanswered Research Questions

As we have noted, in general, women of all ages use more prescription drugs than do men. However, few researchers have done studies to determine why. Five hypotheses have been advanced to account for gender differences in drug use:

☐ It is culturally more acceptable for women to report and medically treat their symptoms.

☐ Women spend more time in the home and thus have easier access to physicians, pharmacists, and the medicine cabinet.

☐ Women's social roles are more dissatisfying, demanding, and/or more stressful.

☐ Women are more likely to be prescribed drugs by health professionals, who perceive them as being more ill or needing more drugs than men.

☐ Women are more likely to have certain types of illnesses, problems, and conditions amenable to drug therapy (e.g., urinary tract infections, hypertension, menopause, etc.)

These are provocative hypotheses, worthy of more extensive investigation. However, to our knowledge, only Dr. Svarstad, of the University of Wisconsin, is exploring these hypotheses in a large community-based sample.

Drug Use and the Elderly in Ambulatory Care Settings: Unanswered Questions

Present knowledge concerning factors affecting drug use in the elderly is derived primarily from studies having methodological flaws. These studies are often based on small populations of volunteers or on other highly selective groups. Low-income, rural, black, and Hispanic elderly are underrepresented. Many of these studies lack control groups of nonelderly respondents, designs are either retrospective or cross-sectional, and patterns of drug use are not examined over time. If we are to understand fully the patterns and dynamics of geriatric drug use, we need more sophisticated studies using multivariate analysis and investigating the effects of long-term drug use.

The studies that we have analyzed have increased our understanding of drug use by the elderly in ambulatory care settings but are limited in several pertinent respects. Most investigators have examined individual factors affecting drug prescribing or drug use. How factors such as age, gender, race, and economic status interact with one another to affect drug use has not been considered. Only a few investigators have employed multivariate statistical techniques to analyze the interrelationship of these variables and their relative importance (Kalimo 1969; Bush & Osterweis 1978). Nor do most studies examine why certain segments of the population use more prescription drugs than do others. For example, nonwhites have somewhat lower rates of drug use than do whites (Gagnon, Salber & Greene 1978). However, for the elderly poor eligible for both Medicare and Medicaid—and this includes a disproportionate percentage of minorities—prescription drug use is higher than for the elderly who are eligible only for Medicare (Wilensky 1983). Thus, effects of illness and third-party payment for physicians' services appear to outweigh cultural factors affecting drug use (Wilensky 1983).

It is also possible that apparent cultural factors are really economic. Nonwhites, mainly black and Hispanic people, are poorer on the average than are whites—a factor that could explain lower drug use. However, Medicaid, in paying for drugs for poor elderly persons, eliminates the economic factor. The generally poorer health of the elderly nonwhite population could account for higher drug use among that population.

Another limitation of many studies examining the use of prescription drugs is their failure to measure drug use over long periods of time. In some studies respondents are asked to specify the drugs that they have taken during the previous two days, two weeks, or two months, but they are not asked to describe their drug use over more extended periods. There are many practical reasons for this lack of longitudinal data. Although investigators have asked respondents to try to recall numbers and types of drugs consumed for as long as a one- to two-year period (May et al. 1982; Stewart, Hale & Marks 1982; Mellinger & Balter 1981), people cannot report reliably the number and types of drugs used over such extended periods. There are more objective and valid methods of measuring long-term use (e.g., reviewing pharmacy records), but they are extremely time-consuming, costly, and difficult to implement on a large-scale basis. Nevertheless, it is essential to obtain longitudinal data if we are to gain a better understanding of the patterns of the elderly's drug use over time—how long individuals take specific drugs, when they start, when they stop, what drugs they substitute, etc. When we have this knowledge, we shall be able to determine why such patterns exist—for example, whether certain patterns are associated with particular subgroups. Most important, we shall know whether health outcomes are affected by specific patterns of drug use.

CHAPTER THREE

Geriatric Drug Misuse and Its Prevention: The Role of the Physician, the Pharmacist, and the Patient

Introduction

E ffective prescription drug therapy depends on rational prescribing by physicians and compliance with drug regimens by patients. Too often, one or both of these critical elements are absent in the care of the elderly. A useful distinction has been made between drug misuse involving errors made by physicians who prescribe, pharmacists who dispense, or nurses who administer prescription drugs inappropriately, and drug misuse involving overuse or underuse of medications, commonly referred to as noncompliance (Maddox 1979). This chapter will deal with the first problem, and the following chapter with the second.

Numerous factors contribute to the problem of geriatric drug misuse. The most serious of these is inappropriate physician prescribing, caused at least in part by an unsatisfactory physician-patient relationship. We will examine geriatric drug misuse in ambulatory care settings, hospitals, and nursing homes, concentrating on the role of the physician and on the physician-patient relationship. We will stress ways to improve physician prescribing, especially methods involving close collaboration with clinical pharmacists.

Like the physician, the pharmacist plays an essential role in assuring appropriate use of prescription and nonprescription drugs by the elderly. However, in the minds of many, pharmacists' activities are still limited to "counting and pouring, licking and sticking." Many health professionals and consumers are unaware of ways in which pharmacists can help ensure safe and effective drug use while simultaneously containing drug costs.

Drug Misuse in Ambulatory Care Settings

Most physician-patient encounters in the United States occur in physicians' private offices. Patients visit physicians not only for acute and chronic illnesses but also for many other reasons, including depression and anxiety, weight problems, sexual problems, loneliness, and other social problems that result in somatic complaints. Most patient visits are return visits; the patient has established an ongoing relationship with a particular physician, and the physician has indicated the need for a return visit. Old patients with old problems (62 percent) and old patients with new problems (23 percent) account for 85 percent of all visits to physicians' offices (U.S. Department of Health, Education, and Welfare 1977b). This continuity creates a framework for a long-term relationship in which both physician and patient can learn to participate in solving or managing the patient's problems.

As we have described in Chapter 2, a number of factors affect physician prescribing. One critical factor in rational prescribing—the physician-patient relationship—is often overlooked (Balint 1964). For example, the deference of many elderly patients toward physicians may cause difficulties. If patients are diffident about communicating their symptoms, concerns, or questions about the use of drugs, symptoms and concerns may be misinterpreted and the wrong drug, or no drug at all, may be prescribed.

Misuse of Psychotropic Medications

Geriatric drug misuse in ambulatory settings extends well beyond problems in physician-patient communication. As discussed in Chapter 2, a crucial drug misuse issue involves the inappropriate prescribing of sedative-hypnotics. In a major study conducted in 1979, the Institute of Medicine was unable to find documentation confirming the efficacy of hypnotics in the elderly. As Miles and Dement point out, "This is a shocking neglect in view of the disproportionate use of sleeping pills by older persons, the age-related changes in drug metabolism, and the much higher incidence of sleep-related respiratory impairment and cardiovascular disease" (Miles & Dement 1980: 190). Since common hypnotic medications, such as chloral hydrate and flurazepam, are more likely to produce side effects in the aged, long-term regimens of sleeping pills should be prescribed with caution.

In addition, elderly Americans are more likely to fall and sustain hip fractures if they use psychotropic drugs, such as antipsychotics, tricyclic antidepressants, and long-acting hypnotic or anxiolytic agents. Nearly 250,000 cases of osteoporotic hip fracture—a leading cause of morbidity and mortality among the elderly—occur each year at a total cost of almost $6 billion.

Previous research has found that psychotropic drugs increase the likelihood of falls among the elderly (Sobel & McCart 1983; Mac-Donald 1984). However, a study by Ray and his colleagues is the first to show a consistent association between the use of a variety of psychotropic drugs and hip fractures in both the institutionalized and noninstitutionalized aged (Ray et al. 1987). Researchers found that Michigan Medicaid enrollees 65 years and older who used an antipsychotic drug were twice as likely to fracture a hip as were nonusers, and that taking a tricyclic antidepressant increased the risk of hip injury by 90 percent. In addition, elderly enrollees using hypnotic or anxiolytic drugs that have long elimination half-lives (i.e., that take the body a day or more to eliminate) had an 80 percent greater chance of breaking a hip than did nonusers. In fact, using higher dosages of psychotropic drugs increased the risk of hip fracture even more. Nearly 14 percent of the hip fractures in the population studied were attributable to falls produced by side effects of psychotropic drugs. If the study findings are confirmed in other populations, it means that a large percentage of all hip fractures among the elderly may be caused indirectly by the use of psychotropic drugs.

The Dangers of Polypharmacy

Another type of medication problem encountered by elderly patients in ambulatory settings involves polypharmacy, or the unnecessary, incorrect, or excessive use of medication. Polypharmacy can take many forms. The problem can involve misuse of nonprescription drugs, of prescription drugs, or of both. Although the term "polypharmacy" is often used in a very broad sense, it can be defined so that it applies to specific problems (Simonson 1984):

☐ Use of medications that have no apparent indication (e.g., prolonged and/or irregular use of sedative-hypnotics for insomnia even though these drugs are frequently ineffective and can potentially exacerbate the insomnia).

☐ Use of duplicate medications—i.e., simultaneous use of different brand-name drugs with similar or identical pharmacologic effects (e.g., use of two different sedative-hypnotics prescribed by two different physicians, producing oversedation, or a "hangover" effect).

☐ Concurrent use of drugs that can result in a drug interaction (e.g., use of antacids with digoxin, thus decreasing absorption of digoxin; use of diuretics with digoxin, causing hypokalemia or low potassium which, if untreated, leads to digoxin toxicity).

☐ Use of contraindicated drugs—i.e., prescribing of medications that are inappropriate for a particular condition (e.g., use of a beta-blocker such as propranolol for patients with heart failure, which can worsen the condition; use of anticoagulants in patients with active peptic ulcer disease).

☐ Use of inappropriate dosages (e.g., excessive doses of the more potent diuretics, which can produce postural hypotension and precipitate falls in the frail elderly).

☐ Use of drugs to treat adverse drug reactions, thus exacerbating the polypharmacy spiral (e.g., use of levodopa to treat Parkinson's-like side effects produced by major tranquilizers).

How widespread is the polypharmacy problem? Although we lack precise data regarding its magnitude, available studies suggest that excessive prescribing is widespread. Why? Many physicians do not recognize that the elderly are especially susceptible to drug-related problems because of age-related changes in the body's mechanisms of drug distribution, metabolism, and excretion (Lamy 1980). Consequently, commonly used drugs such as digoxin and cimetidine are frequently prescribed in dosages excessive for elderly patients (Whiting, Wandless & Sumner 1978; Manning et al. 1980; Campion et al. 1985).

There is also the more insidious problem of side effects that go "undetected, untreated, and unexplained" by physicians (McKenney et al. 1973). These side effects often result from ingestion of many different kinds of medications concurrently and contribute to more serious adverse drug reactions. For example, one of the most common causes of reversible dementia is the injudicious use of medications (Kane, Ouslander & Abrass 1984; Beck et al. 1982).

Undermedication

Overmedication is often seen as the major drug misuse problem plaguing the noninstitutionalized elderly, but undermedication may be an equally serious and frequently overlooked phenomenon. Chronic illnesses afflicting the elderly—depression, arthritis, diabetes mellitus, and osteoporosis—may be undertreated by physicians. Physicians may fail to prescribe needed drugs or may prescribe them in less than adequate amounts for a less than adequate period of time. One area in which undermedication is apparent and potentially serious is in the treatment of depression. Physicians may fail to treat depression in elderly patients because it can exhibit atypical symptoms (e.g., mental confusion). When it is correctly identified, it may not be treated at all, for physicians may consider depression an inherent part of the aging process. Even when antidepressant drug therapy is initiated, dosages may be too low because physicians either are overly cautious or are unaware of the availability of a wide variety of antidepressant drugs with differing side-effect profiles. Such variety permits physicians to individualize therapy by monitoring blood levels (Task Force on Use of Laboratory Tests in Psychiatry 1985).

Another instance of undermedication can be observed in the use of chemotherapeutic agents for cancer. Geriatric patients often are omitted from chemotherapeutic treatment for fear that they will develop life-threatening toxicities. When they are placed on chemotherapeutic treatment, clinicians may assume that the dosages of these drugs should be reduced because of the potential for serious adverse drug reactions. In fact, recent evidence suggests that in order to produce any therapeutic effect in older adults, these agents must be given in full dosages (Kelly 1986).

Consequences of Inappropriate Physician Prescribing

Less than optimal physician prescribing can result in hospitalization for the elderly. It is estimated that up to 10 percent of hospital admissions and readmissions may be caused by adverse drug reactions, which are often a result of inappropriate prescribing. Geriatric patients are especially at risk (Hurwitz 1969b; Learoyd 1972; Wynne & Heller 1973; Williamson 1979). Drugs most frequently implicated in such admissions include anticonvulsants, antidiabetics, antihypertensives, anti-Parkinsonian agents, corticosteroids, cardiovascular agents, and tranquilizers (Caranasos, Stewart & Cluff 1974; McKenney & Harrison 1976; Bergman & Wiholm 1981; Hurwitz 1969b; Williamson 1979). Not all drug-related hospitalizations are preventable. Some are unavoidable reactions produced by the prescribing of necessary drugs in appropriate dosages. However, hospitalizations that result from inappropriate dosages, avoidable drug-drug interactions, or physicians' lack of awareness of the increased toxicity of many drugs in the elderly *are* preventable.

Drug Misuse in Hospitals

Prescription drug use in hospitals represents a potentially more serious problem than it does in ambulatory care settings because patients are sicker and often require multiple therapies simultaneously. Numerous studies have described the extent of misuse of prescription drugs among patients of all ages in hospitals. For example, studies performed more than a decade ago reported misuse of antibiotics in community, university, and Veterans Administration hospitals. Antimicrobial agents were administered when they were not needed at all; inappropriate antibiotics or dosages were used in 30 to 60 percent of all treated patients; and prophylactic antibiotics were continued beyond the necessary or appropriate period to achieve the desired therapeutic outcome (Craig 1978; Castle et al. 1977; Maki & Schuna 1978; Hoffman 1978; Lee 1979). Misuse, however, is not limited to antibiotics.

In analyzing research relating to drug use among hospitalized patients, Soumerai and Avorn (1984) found ample evidence of inappropriate prescribing:

☐ Use of a potentially toxic drug when one with less risk of toxicity would work as well (e.g., the use of phenylbutazone in patients with osteoarthritis or rheumatoid arthritis when other nonsteroidal anti-inflammatory drugs would be less hazardous).

☐ Use of the wrong drug for a given indication (e.g., phenobarbital for disturbances of sleep in a patient who is a heavy drinker).

☐ Concurrent administration of an excessive number of drugs, which increases the possibility of interaction effects (a special risk for the elderly, many of whom suffer from multiple chronic illnesses).

☐ Excessive doses, especially for elderly patients (e.g., digoxin).

☐ Continued use of a drug after evidence becomes available concerning major toxic or even lethal side effects (e.g., chloramphenicol).

The most serious consequence of inappropriate prescribing in hospitals is an increase in the number and severity of adverse drug reactions (Chapter 1). Less well documented, but of considerable consequence, is the avoidable morbidity and mortality caused by physicians' failure to provide effective drugs for treatable diseases.

In addition to direct medical consequences, inappropriate drug prescribing in hospitals results in major unnecessary costs. Limited health care resources are wasted when expensive drugs are used if less costly products would be equally effective, when unnecessary drugs are prescribed, or when medications are continued beyond pharmacologic need (Soumerai & Avorn 1984).

Inappropriate drug prescribing is most likely to occur when physicians fail to review medication orders frequently and critically and when they are unable to keep abreast of rapid developments in pharmacology and therapeutics. Lack of communication between pharmacist and physician can further aggravate the problem.

Drug-related problems for hospitalized elderly patients are particularly acute. The severity and complexity of the conditions suffered by older people often require the use of multiple drugs, of potentially toxic drugs, and of drugs in which the difference between a therapeutic and a toxic dose is small (e.g., digoxin or warfarin).

Undermedication in Hospitals: The Care of the Terminally Ill

Physicians frequently underutilize pain medication for terminally ill patients, many of whom are elderly. Every day, thousands of patients suffer unnecessarily because a drug is administered in inadequate doses or over excessively long intervals (Rial 1983). The hospice philosophy of regularly scheduled oral administration of narcotic analgesics, while gaining credibility, has not been fully accepted by physicians and nurses (Marks & Sachar 1973). In an evaluation of the quality of care provided to hospitalized terminally ill patients, poor pain management was cited as a significant problem in 60 percent of the terminal cases rated as receiving poor quality care (Loomis & Williams 1983).

The reasons for inadequate pain control are complex. Patients are often reluctant to reveal the severity of their pain or to take narcotics. Relatives often have misguided concerns that the terminally ill patient will develop a drug dependence. Physicians and nurses may be reluctant to prescribe and administer round-the-clock doses of potent analgesics because of inadequate pharmacologic knowledge, misconceptions regarding addiction liability, and fear of death (Reuler, Girard & Nardone 1980; Health and Public Policy Committee 1983).

Drug Misuse in Nursing Homes

A major area of drug use and misuse among the aged is in skilled nursing and intermediate care facilities. There are, at present, more nursing home beds than acute care beds in the United States. Currently 1.5 million elderly patients reside in nursing homes, and their number is expected to increase as the number of elderly, particularly those over age 75, increases. While only 5 percent of the elderly are in nursing homes, 22 percent of those 85 years and over are in nursing homes, and about 1 in 5 older Americans will spend some time living in such institutions (Rice & Feldman 1983). As we have mentioned, estimates suggest that drugs are dispensed regularly to over 95 percent of the elderly who reside in nursing homes (Cooper 1981).

In 1976 a research team in the Office of Long-Term Care, Department of Health, Education, and Welfare (DHEW) surveyed 1,731,360 drug orders issued in 288 skilled nursing facilities. Seventy-eight percent of the patients in these facilities were 65 years of age or over. The DHEW team concluded that in skilled nursing facilities multiple drug prescribing for individual patients is the prevailing pattern (U.S. Department of Health, Education, and Welfare 1976). The average number of prescriptions issued per patient per day was 6.1, and the total number of prescriptions per patient ranged from 0 to 23 per day. Drugs tended to be prescribed to alleviate symptoms rather than for strictly therapeutic purposes. Cathartics were the single largest class prescribed (53 percent of patients), followed by analgesics (48 percent) and tranquilizers (45 percent). Sedatives and hypnotics were prescribed to one-third of the patients (see Table 3.1).

Psychotropic drugs present the greatest potential for misuse in nursing homes (U.S. Senate 1975; Cooper 1978). Psychotropic drugs are among those most frequently prescribed and administered in nursing homes, and they present significant costs and risks to the elderly persons receiving them. The institutionalized aged spend seventeen times more on psychotropic drugs than do the noninstitutionalized aged (Zadawski, Glazer & Lurie 1978).

About one-half of all nursing home residents take some form of tranquilizer. Residents often receive sedatives on a nightly basis for extended periods of time, and a considerable number of these residents experience adverse reactions (e.g., mental confusion) from chronic use (Marttila et al. 1977). Because they can decrease alertness, affect judgment and balance, and cause dizziness, sedative-hypnotics

TABLE 3.1

Number and Percent of Patients Receiving Drugs by Drug Category in Rank Order
in a 250,000 Patient Skilled Nursing Facility Population

	Patients		
Drug categories	Number	Percent	Rank
Cathartics	1,839	53.3%	1
Analgesics and antipyretics	1,645	47.7	2
Tranquilizers	1,549	44.8	3
Other	1,258	36.4	4
Diuretics	1,169	33.8	5
Vitamins	1,149	33.3	6
Sedatives and hypnotics	1,147	33.2	7
Cardiac drugs	1,000	28.9	8
Skin and mucous membranes	613	17.7	9
Antiinfectives	539	16.9	10
Antacids and absorbents	489	14.2	11
Antihistamines	479	13.8	12
Hypotensives	428	12.4	13
Eye, ear, nose, and throat	408	11.8	14
Spasmolytics	394	11.4	15
Insulin and antidiabetic agents	384	11.1	16
Controlled substances (Schedule II)	372	10.7	17
Electrolyte replacement	345	9.9	18
Vasodilating agents	298	8.5	19
Antidepressants	289	8.4	20
Anticonvulsants	257	7.4	21
Estrogens/androgens	212	3.5	22
Thyroid replacements[a]	87	2.5	23
Adrenals	77	2.2	24
Anticoagulants	37	1.0	25

SOURCE: American Society of Hospital Pharmacists Formulary Service, Washington, D.C.
Adapted from Long-Term Care Facility Improvement Study: Introductory Report, U.S. Dept. of
HEW, Office of Nursing Home Affairs, July 1975: 52.
[a] Includes antithyroid agents.

contribute to an increased risk of falls among elderly nursing home
residents (Sobel & McCart 1983). Such falls can lead to hip and verte-
bral fractures, with accompanying morbidity and mortality (Mac-
Donald & MacDonald 1977; Ray et al. 1987). Other drugs routinely
given to nursing home residents—major tranquilizers, tricyclic antidepressants, antihypertensives and diuretics—are also suspected of
causing falls because of effects similar to those of sedative-hypnotics
(MacDonald 1984; Sobel & McCart 1983).

In a major study involving review of 384,326 prescriptions for patients 65 years and older in 173 Tennessee nursing homes, researchers found that psychotropic drugs, particularly antipsychotics, were prescribed far more frequently than they were for a group of noninstitutionalized Medicaid recipients with the same sociodemographic characteristics (Ray, Federspiel & Schaffner 1980). In one year an average of 67 prescriptions per person were dispensed to the nursing home patients, whereas the ambulatory patients received an average of 30 prescriptions. Seventy-four percent of the nursing home residents were prescribed psychotropic drugs; of the ambulatory patients, only 36 percent received such prescriptions. Antipsychotic drugs were the most common psychotropic drug prescribed in nursing homes; 43 percent of the nursing home patients received them, compared with 10 percent of the ambulatory group.

The Tennessee study found extraordinary variation in antipsychotic drug use among nursing homes. In 43 nursing homes (25 percent of the sample), none of the patients was a chronic recipient of antipsychotic drugs, whereas in 15 homes (less than 10 percent of the sample) 20 to 46 percent of the patients received such drugs on a regular basis. The authors tried to account for such disparities by examining characteristics of the nursing homes. They looked at factors such as availability of institutional resources for patient care, violations of state licensing requirements, and ratings resulting from elaborate, expensive, federally required inspections of the facilities. None of these factors was predictive. However, chronic use of antipsychotic drugs correlated positively with the size of the nursing home and correlated negatively with the staff-per-patient ratio. These correlations suggest that antipsychotic drugs may be used in large institutions as a substitute for personnel.

There also was wide variation in physicians' prescribing of antipsychotic drugs. In the Tennessee study a small group of family practitioners, 50 percent of whom practiced in rural counties, prescribed most of the antipsychotic medications. As physicians' nursing home practice increased in size (more patients in more nursing homes), physicians prescribed increasing amounts of antipsychotic drugs per patient. Physicians graduating between 1950 and 1959 were most likely to prescribe these drugs. This was the decade when chlorpromazine, a major tranquilizer, was first introduced and when psychotropic drug use became widespread.

Despite increased concern about the magnitude, appropriateness, and cost of psychotropic drug use in nursing homes, there is insufficient understanding of the reasons for this use. We do not know whether physicians, nurses, or others initiate prescriptions for psychotropic drugs. Nor do we know the factors that determine physicians' decisions to authorize psychotropic medications or that affect nurses' decisions to administer them. The impact that nurses have on use of these drugs has not been closely examined. This is particularly surprising, for about one-half of the drugs in nursing homes are prescribed on a PRN or "as needed" basis. Nurses' role in suggesting psychotropic drugs to patients' physicians and their readiness to administer these drugs are two important and relatively unexplored areas in which research is needed.

How can we explain the finding that the elderly in nursing homes receive far more psychotropic medications than do the noninstitutionalized elderly? A number of hypotheses may be considered:

☐ The process of institutionalization, along with removal from familiar surroundings and friends, is so disorienting for patients that they need or demand psychotropic drugs.

☐ Elderly patients who are most in need of psychotropic medications are those most likely to be placed in nursing homes.

☐ The lack of widely accepted, clear-cut medical guidelines for the prescribing of these drugs leads physicians to use them more often than is clinically indicated.

☐ Nursing home patients insist on psychotropic agents, particularly tranquilizers and sedatives, because they are already accustomed to using them.

☐ Excessive amounts of psychotropic drugs are given to nursing home residents to keep the wards quiet and reduce the number of staff required to care for patients. (This explanation—drugs used as "chemical straitjackets"—is the one most commonly offered.)

☐ The attitudes, knowledge, and status of nurses play a critical role, especially their attitudes toward the elderly and their belief in the value of psychotropic drugs.

It is possible that different forces are at work in different kinds of settings. For example, some studies have concluded that proprietary nursing homes are associated with lower quality of care than are nonprofit facilities (Vladeck 1980). The relationship between nursing home ownership and psychotropic drug use raises unanswered questions. Indeed, the entire issue of widespread use of psychotropic drugs in nursing homes is a matter of extreme concern for all physicians and for other health professionals responsible for the care of patients in these settings. If these problems are to be illuminated and redressed, additional research is needed.

Undermedication in Nursing Homes

In addition to the problem of overmedication, there is some evidence that undermedication also may be occurring, though its extent and causes are unknown. For example, a General Accounting Office review of one month's records of 106 Medicaid patients in fourteen nursing homes in California showed that 311 drug doses were given in amounts larger than had been ordered by physicians, but 1,210 prescribed doses had not been administered at all (U.S. General Accounting Office 1970). Unfortunately, the types of drugs least likely to be administered were not specified in the report. Nor were any explanations offered for the undermedication. Several factors could, however, have been responsible: nurses' judgments about the appropriateness of the prescriptions, understaffing, high staff turnover, unskilled and ill-informed staff, and nurses' and/or aides' attitudes toward the aged. Although clinical outcomes were not examined, the effects of undermedication on patients' health may have been quite serious.

The only study to investigate clinicians' treatment decisions in nursing homes, conducted by Brown and Thompson in 1979, examined decisions not to treat febrile patients. Results revealed that 57 percent of the patients received active treatment (antibiotics, hospitalization, or both), whereas 43 percent received no treatment. Factors showing a significant relation to nontreatment included diagnosis (patients with cancer showed the highest incidence of nontreatment); mental status of the patient (patients who were comatose were less likely to be treated); mobility (patients who were bedridden were less likely to be treated); pain (patients in pain were less likely to be treated); narcotics prescribed (patients receiving narcotics were less likely to be treated); size of the facility (smaller facilities were associated with nontreatment); physician's specialty (patients whose primary physicians were oncologists or surgeons were less likely to be treated); and medical-record statements documenting the patient's deterioration or plans for nontreatment because of, for example, irreversible life-threatening conditions (patients whose conditions were described as deteriorating and patients whose medical records indicated plans for nontreatment were more likely not to be treated). These relationships suggest that patients whose medical condition was terminal and whose quality of life was poor were less likely to receive active treatment for their fevers and that the nontreatment decision was deliberate and appropriate.

It is important to note, however, that not all of the patients with these characteristics were untreated. Furthermore, many patients who did not have these characteristics were untreated. The results raise serious questions. Why was no treatment given to one-fourth of the patients whose medical records contained no evidence of terminal status or poor prognosis? Why was no treatment given to over one-third of the patients whose records revealed no plans to limit treatment? Poor charting practices may provide part of the answer, but questions still remain. It might be argued that it is appropriate and humane not to treat certain acute infections in patients with terminal illnesses or other advanced and irreversible life-threatening conditions. However, nontreatment of patients whose medical conditions are stable seems far less justifiable.

The Role of the Physician in Drug Use

Physicians' Perceptions of the Elderly

We have considered how drugs are prescribed and administered to the elderly in a variety of settings, but it is also important to examine how physicians' perceptions of the elderly may influence drug misuse and its prevention. The results of one study showed that physician-patient encounter time declined as a function of age. This decline was observed for eight out of nine kinds of physicians studied, across the range of primary problem severity and regardless of the type of encounter (Kane et al. 1980b; Keeler et al. 1982). The researchers suggested that decreased encounter time for the elderly may result, in part, from physicians' perceptions that aged persons are not priority patients. A lack of awareness of ways to observe and measure progress in elderly patients may also aggravate negative attitudes. Furthermore, inadequate time spent with these patients may affect the quality of physicians' diagnoses and prescribing.

Studies have compared the attitudes of medical students toward the elderly at the start and end of their training. The studies show that, in general, there is deterioration in students' attitudes toward elderly patients and in their desire to care for them (Gale & Livesley 1974; Spence et al. 1968).

The attitudes of practicing physicians also appear to be less than optimal. A study of physicians' attitudes toward the aged in nursing homes found that physicians expressed a definite lack of interest in the care of such patients. Almost 40 percent of the physicians in the study viewed the nursing home as a place to die, and 25 percent considered treatment of patients over 75 years of age as less challenging than treatment of younger patients (Miller et al. 1976).

A study of age as a factor in evaluation and treatment of adult psychiatric outpatients reported similar findings (Karasu et al. 1979). A comparison of therapist ratings and patient self-ratings in three age groups found that patients 42 to 64 years of age were seen as sicker, but less treatable, than younger patients or patients in the same age group as the therapist. Therapists expressed a decided preference for treating those patients who were under 42 years of age. The therapists thought that motivation for treatment, prognosis, and capacity for insights were more favorable in the younger age groups. Patients 65 years of age and older were not treated in the clinic under study and therefore were not included in the analysis; however, it is reasonable to assume that therapists' attitudes toward age applied to this older age group as well. The researchers concluded that greater attention should be directed toward the ages of the patient and the therapist as often unrecognized but critical factors in patient evaluation, selection for treatment, and therapeutic outcome.

An analysis of the portrayal of the elderly and nonelderly in prescription drug advertisements in two medical journals revealed that, in a majority of advertisements, both types of patients were presented in a negative way but that the unfavorable portrayal of the elderly tended to reinforce invidious societal stereotypes about them. Because commercial messages often have a strong impact, these advertisements may predispose physicians to negative viewpoints of the elderly and adversely influence the quality of their drug prescribing (Smith 1976).

Physician-Patient Relationships

Physicians' perceptions of the elderly are only one of the factors that can affect physician prescribing. The physician-patient relationship, a complex interaction, is another critically important factor. Traditional models used to explain the interaction between patients and physicians emphasize the passivity of the patient and the power of the physician (Parsons 1951). In their classic article Szasz and Hollender (1956) conceptualized three models of physician-patient relations: (1) the activity-passivity model, (2) the guidance-cooperation model, and (3) the mutual participation model. Each of these relationships is appropriate under different circumstances.

The activity-passivity model operates when the physician is active and the patient is passive. The physician assumes a role similar to that of parent, and the patient the role of helpless infant (Szasz & Hollender 1956). Sometimes the patient is simply unable to participate, and treatment proceeds without the patient's contribution (e.g., when a patient is in a coma, is undergoing emergency care for severe injuries, or is undergoing surgery). Under these conditions, patient compliance with prescribed drugs does not constitute a problem, because drugs are administered either directly by a physician or under supervision of a nurse.

At other times, however, the activity-passivity model may be inappropriate. The patient may be able but unwilling to assume an active role, because he or she believes that physicians are authorities and have the right to make medical decisions and that patients are obligated to obey. Under these conditions, compliance could constitute a problem, because patients who are dissatisfied with their drug regimen might be unwilling to question their physicians for fear of challenging physician authority. This attitude could lead to "hidden" noncompliance, ultimately compromising therapeutic outcome. The prescribing physician, unaware of the patient's lack of compliance, may attribute changes in the patient's health to the prescribed therapy rather than to other factors, such as the course of the disease, diagnostic error, or effects of concomitant therapy. Such incorrect attributions could lead to inappropriate changes in prescribing and, ultimately, a decline in the patient's health.

The guidance-cooperation model, in which the patient assumes a more active role, has been described by Szasz and Hollender as similar to a parent-child or parent-adolescent relationship. When a patient is in the early stages of recovery from a heart attack or has a severe infection, he or she is usually capable of following instructions and exercising some judgment, but the physician makes the decisions. The patient is expected to "look up to" and "obey" the physician without questioning the "orders" received.

In a third kind of relationship both physician and patient participate actively. When the patient is willing and able to take much of the responsibility for his or her treatment and the physician helps the patient to achieve this objective, the relationship is one of mutual participation—an adult-to-adult relationship (Szasz & Hollender 1956). This type of relationship is realistic—even necessary—in the management of most chronic conditions (e.g., diabetes mellitus, chronic heart disease, hypertension, etc.). Here the patient's own experiences provide reliable and important clues for therapy. Also, the treatment program is carried out principally by the patient. In 1956, when Szasz and Hollender first introduced this model of the physician-patient relationship, it was described as "foreign to medical practice." Today, however, consumer activists and others involved in health care have urged that this type of relationship become typical. Some health professionals argue that mutual participation by patients and physicians is increasingly necessary, particularly for the elderly, because of the growing emphasis on management of chronic disease rather than care of acute illness.

Mutual Participation by Physician and Patient: Rhetoric Versus Reality

Traditional types of physician-patient relationships are based upon trust between patient and physician and compliance with the physician's instructions. These old models, however, are being challenged by consumer health advocates, activists in the women's health movement, the self-care movement, organized groups of elderly (e.g., Gray Panthers, American Association of Retired Persons), and individual patients wishing to become more involved in their own care. New physician-patient relationships may be based on adult-to-adult communication, sometimes involving confrontation and conflict. Patients may confront and challenge physicians with demands for detailed information that physicians may not be able or willing to provide. Patients may also demand that their rights be recognized, including the right to refuse treatment. These changes in physician-patient relationships are also connected to the impact that the consumer movement is having on the policies of the Food and Drug Administration with respect to the labeling of prescription drugs—a subject that will be discussed in Chapter 8.

Despite rhetoric about and trends toward more active patient involvement, studies suggest that traditional relationships—active-passive and guidance-cooperation models—still hold in most cases, including those involving elderly patients and their physicians (Haug 1979; Lipton & Svarstad 1974; Svarstad 1976). It is entirely possible that mutual participation may not be desired by or be appropriate for all elderly patients. In fact, the present generation of elderly might be more comfortable with the familiar activity-passivity or guidance-cooperation models. There is information to support this view. Data obtained from interviews in a survey of 640 persons revealed that respondents aged 60 years and over are more likely to accept physician authority than are younger people (Haug 1979). In contrast, future generations of the elderly are likely to be better educated and more sophisticated medically. As a result, physicians working with the elderly of the future may have to exercise less traditional authority in encounters with patients and rely more on a relationship based on mutual participation.

It is difficult to determine what would actually happen if the tables were turned and patients participated fully. Little is known, for example, about patients' influence on physician prescribing. The early work of Freidson (1960) on client control suggests that the institution-bound elderly may be able to exercise less control in the physician-patient relationship than can patients in less supervised settings. The nature, extent, and consequences of patient pressure in ambulatory settings have been explored in at least one study. The results indicate that this phenomenon can indeed compromise physicians' therapeutic decisions (Podell, Kent & Keller 1976). Anecdotally, many practicing physicians have observed that patients request, and in some cases demand, specific drug therapies that may be contraindicated (e.g., an antibiotic for a common cold, a particular hypertensive said by friends to be effective, long-term use of minor tranquilizers to cope with stressful situations, or vitamins and tonics to combat fatigue). To what extent and under what circumstances do elderly patients demand drugs that are inappropriate? To what extent do physicians succumb to these demands, and with what consequences for the course and outcome of treatment? The influence of patient expectations and pressures on the quality of physician prescribing needs to be clarified.

The Growing Role of the Clinical Pharmacist in Drug Use

To understand the contribution that today's pharmacist can make, it is important to appreciate the dramatic changes that have taken place in pharmacy education. During the past two decades, "clinical" pharmacists—pharmacists who are patient-oriented as opposed to product-oriented—have significantly expanded their professional responsibilities. Such pharmacists now assess drug response, identify adverse drug effects and drug-drug interactions, provide drug consultations to physicians, and improve patient compliance by educating patients and monitoring drug therapy (Stimmel & McGhan 1981; Lee 1979). Half of the nation's seventy-three pharmacy schools have Doctor of Pharmacy (Pharm.D.) programs that prepare pharmacists for these expanded clinical roles. Graduate-level programs generally provide two years or more of training beyond the baccalaureate degree (Covington 1983).

A growing literature supports the idea that clinical pharmacists can enhance physicians' drug therapy decisions, improve patient compliance, curtail drug costs, and reduce outpatient visits and hospitalizations (Bond & Salinger 1979; Sczupak & Conrad 1977; Hood & Murphy 1978). These outcomes have been demonstrated in teaching hospitals (Keys, South & Duffy 1975; Brooks et al. 1977; Herfindal, Bernstein & Kishi 1983), in outpatient settings (McKenney et al. 1973; McKenney et al. 1978; Rosen & Holmes 1978), in home-based populations (Hammarlund et al. 1985), and in skilled nursing facilities (Cheung & Kayne 1975; Strandberg et al. 1980). In nursing home settings pharmacists are required by federal regulations to review, at least monthly, the records of all Medicare patients (Federal Register 1974). Although the federal regulations have had a positive impact on drug use in many nursing homes, they have not produced uniform results. Nor can this level of intermittent participation by pharmacists correct the serious deficiencies in drug prescribing and management that currently exist in most nursing homes.

In addition to these consultative roles, pharmacists' functions have been expanded to include drug prescribing under physician supervision, a new function tested in an innovative experiment begun in California. In 1977 California became the first state in the nation to permit the formation of special projects in which clinical pharmacists, nurse practitioners, and physicians' assistants could prescribe and dispense medications under physician supervision (Stimmel & McGhan 1981). Similar legislation expanding the clinical pharmacist's role was subsequently enacted in Washington and Oregon (Covington 1983).

A great deal of research was done to assess the impact of the pharmacist serving as prescriber. About sixty pharmacists with Doctor of Pharmacy degrees participated in the two California programs, one based in the School of Pharmacy at the University of California at San Francisco (UCSF) and the other in the School of Pharmacy at the University of Southern California (USC) in Los Angeles. The pharmacists worked in diverse health care settings, concentrating on patients with chronic diseases. Researchers evaluated the prescribing of pharmacists who worked at a Kaiser Mental Health Center (Stimmel et al. 1982) and a Kaiser Medical Center (McGhan et al. 1983). Results indicated that specially trained pharmacists prescribe for ambulatory patients at least as well as do physicians.

Of more relevance to the specific health problems of the elderly are results of a study conducted in a skilled nursing facility in which clinical pharmacists, working under a physician's supervision, assessed patients' needs, ordered laboratory tests, and prescribed drugs. The results after one year were dramatic: the number of drugs used monthly for each patient monitored by a clinical pharmacist declined, on the average, from eight to six. Compared with the control group, made up of patients receiving traditional care from physicians, the group receiving prescriptions from clinical pharmacists had a significantly lower number of deaths. Although the number of patient discharges was small, the discharge rate climbed 400 percent; patients seen by pharmacists and physicians working together were more likely to be discharged to a lower level of care (e.g., intermediate care facility or home) than were patients seen by physicians alone. Decreasing the number of drugs per patient, reducing the hospitalization rate, and discharging patients to lower levels of care could result in substantial cost savings. The authors of the study estimated that intervention has the potential for saving the health care system approximately $70,000 per year per 100 skilled nursing facility beds (Thompson et al. 1984).

Strategies for Action

Encouraging Appropriate Drug Use in Ambulatory Settings

Several studies described earlier have suggested that some physicians have negative attitudes toward elderly patients and that these attitudes may compromise quality of care, including drug therapy. The studies cited emphasize the need for increased training of physicians and other health professionals on issues relating to age. Because negative perceptions of the elderly are part of a larger set of cultural attitudes toward aging, better education of health professionals about the needs, abilities, limitations, and potential of the elderly is perhaps the best way to improve attitudes and quality of care (Pfeiffer 1979).

Perhaps the most challenging task in the treatment of elderly patients with chronic illness involves the development of collaborative physician-patient relationships, with active participation by patients in the management of their own drug therapies. Patients have a right and a need to know as much as possible about the drugs they take— why these drugs are prescribed and how they should be taken. Physicians must know when patients discontinue drug treatment or modify the drug regimen. Further, physicians have an obligation to monitor patients' drug therapy in both acute and chronic illness, to be aware of both prescription and nonprescription drug use, to look for signs of adverse reactions or other troublesome side effects, and to be alert to problems of noncompliance. Achieving the goal of rational, appropriate, effective drug therapy is not easy. It requires, at minimum, an open and honest relationship between physician and patient.

Encouraging Appropriate Use of Psychotropic Medications

In order to decrease the use of sedative-hypnotics by the elderly, researchers have explored short-term nonpharmacological approaches to sleep disorders (Coates & Thoreson 1982). Such approaches include, for example, regular exercise, stimulus control instructions,* or training in relaxation skills combined with instruction in problem solving and self-management. These procedures hold considerable promise for the successful treatment of sleep disturbances among the elderly (Bootzin & Engle-Friedman 1987). While not all older persons may be receptive to such approaches, physicians should consider giving patients these choices.

Physicians' abilities to prescribe psychotropic drugs appropriately will be greatly aided by more drug epidemiology studies, such as the one conducted by Ray and associates cited earlier in the chapter. Large-scale studies of this nature—linking patterns of prescribing to

---

*Stimulus control instructions involve a set of specific behavioral rules designed to help insomniacs acquire consistent sleep rhythms.

clinical outcomes, both good and bad—will make important contributions to safe and effective prescribing of psychotropic agents.

Dealing with the Problem of Polypharmacy

The problem of polypharmacy can be addressed if primary physicians become good medical managers. Physicians must be aware of the patient's overall drug regimen, including drugs prescribed by other physicians (e.g., subspecialists) and any nonprescription drugs taken by the patient. Then they must screen out unnecessary or duplicate drugs. Physicians should undertake a periodic review to determine whether a drug regimen is still appropriate, whether it is helping to improve the patient's condition, and whether it is causing any adverse reactions. The latter is particularly important because the elderly experience more adverse drug reactions than do younger persons. Since the risk of these reactions increases with the number of drugs taken, physicians should carefully monitor patients who take multiple medications. Physicians must also be aware that interactions can occur not only between medications but also between medications and food.

In elderly patients interactions often are symptomatically minor. The consequences, however, can sometimes be serious and even lethal. Obviously, it may be difficult for physicians to familiarize themselves with all but the most commonly occurring drug interactions. However, it is possible to use computer programs along with ongoing feedback from clinical pharmacists to help reduce the risk of adverse drug reactions.

One exciting and innovative approach to improving physicians' prescribing involves the public-interest detailer—a physician or pharmacist sponsored by a medical school or medical society. The public-interest detailer provides physicians with up-to-date and unbiased information about drug therapy. (Public-interest detailing will be discussed in Chapter 7.)

Encouraging Appropriate Drug Prescribing in Hospitals

Physician Education

Problems associated with physician prescribing in hospitals were described earlier. These included overmedication, errors of omission, ignorance or disregard of cost factors, inadequate review of medication orders, and lack of information about new developments in pharmacology. Strategies to overcome these problems have been developed and evaluated in several studies. All of these studies suggest that one-to-one education of physicians by drug therapy experts (physicians or pharmacists) is the most effective way to improve physicians' prescribing.

In addition, these educational efforts must be ongoing. A comprehensive review of interventions designed to improve physician prescribing in hospitals concluded that none of the effective interventions produced effects that lasted after the experimental programs were discontinued (Soumerai & Avorn 1984). In other words, ongoing reinforcement was necessary to maintain results. Interestingly, ongoing reinforcement also emerges as an important factor in maintaining elderly patients' compliance with prescribed drug therapy.

Although these studies have similar results, all have limitations. Many lack well-controlled research designs. Data on the economic costs and benefits of educating physicians in drug therapy are often missing. Few studies do cost-effectiveness analyses to determine whether the savings justify the monies expended to mount and maintain the programs. Finally, patients' clinical outcomes—ultimately, the most important measure of physician performance—are not always evaluated.

The Impact of the Diagnosis Related Group (DRG) System on Drug Prescribing in Hospitals

The Health Care Financing Administration (HCFA) regulations adopted in 1983 established a hospital prospective payment system for Medicare patients that is likely to have an impact on drug prescribing for hospitalized Medicare patients. The prospective system of payment provides a fixed payment to hospitals per discharge. The method of determining such payments has been based on the diagnosis related group (DRG)* method. The DRG system offers incentives to hospitals to reduce both the length of stay of Medicare pa-

---

*DRGs classify cases encountered in hospital acute care into clinically coherent groups, which are reasonably similar in hospital resource use and cost. The groups reflect not only a patient's principal diagnosis but also comorbidity and complicating conditions, surgical procedures performed, and the patient's age, sex, and discharge status. There are about 470 DRG groups.

tients and the resources used for their care, including drugs. It is difficult to predict the long-term effects of the DRG payment system. However, in its first two years it has already contributed, nationwide, to a 16 percent reduction in length of stay—from 10 days in fiscal year 1983 to 8.4 days in fiscal year 1985 (Beebe, Callahan & Mariano 1986). In the same two-year period there has been an 11.5 percent reduction in the number of hospital admissions (U.S. Department of Health and Human Services, Health Care Financing Administration, Bureau of Data Management and Strategy, Office of Statistics and Data Management 1987).

State policies regarding hospital payment are also being rapidly modified to achieve more effective hospital cost containment. Whereas some states have followed HCFA's lead and have adopted in their state Medicaid programs new prospective payment policies that follow the DRG system, others have adopted prospective payment systems based on a negotiated rate per day. Still others have adopted more sweeping regulatory reforms, such as mandatory hospital rate-setting policies, based on per diem rate limits or global budgets for hospitals. The overall effect of most of these changes will be to reduce incentives for physicians to prescribe large numbers of drugs in hospitals.

First, hospitals will probably institute more rigorous programs of drug utilization review and will probably use restrictive measures, such as formularies, to reduce prescription drug use. Second, hospitals may also require more stringent and pervasive quality assurance and utilization measures, some of which will concern prescription drugs. These measures will make it easier to monitor use and to evaluate the effectiveness of controls. Third, because of the DRG system, hospitals probably will focus not only on utilization of drugs but also on costs. Recently, for example, the Antibiotic Advisory Subcommittee of the Pharmacy and Therapeutics Committee, made up of clinical pharmacy and medical faculty of the UCSF Medical Center, devoted an entire newsletter to the comparative costs of antibiotics. Noting that antibiotics account for 30 percent of all inpatient drug expenditures at UCSF Medical Center, the subcommittee compared costs of different antibiotics in the treatment of seven different infections. There were dramatic differences in the cost of treating specific infections with different antibiotic agents (Guglielmo et al. 1986).

Despite favorable signs, we cannot be absolutely certain that the quality and economy of drug prescribing will improve under DRGs.

The hospital utilization review policies for Medicare that are now required by HCFA add an extra layer of review in the form of an external peer review organization (PRO). Because the PROs must operate under performance-based contracts, they must meet agreed-upon goals for the reduction of hospital utilization by Medicare beneficiaries. The control given PROs is already causing problems for some hospitals. Tensions may result between the criteria adopted by the external PRO and those used by the hospital's internal quality review. Further, it is possible that patients' reduced length of hospital stay under DRGs may result in less opportunity to stabilize drug therapy and monitor adverse drug effects during hospitalization, leading in turn to increased drug therapy problems after discharge. Clearly, there is need for comprehensive research documenting the full impact of DRGs on drug therapy.

Appropriate Prescribing in Nursing Homes

Physician-Pharmacist Cooperation: The Pharmacist as Prescriber Under Physician Supervision

Perhaps the greatest need for close cooperation among health professionals is in the care of the elderly in nursing homes, settings in which problems of drug misuse are prevalent. The California experiment described earlier, especially that aspect permitting pharmacists to prescribe in institutional settings, provides one model that can be used for widespread testing.

The final report of the California project indicated a cost savings of almost $3 million a year for the 500,000 persons who received services from nonphysician professionals (California Office of Statewide Health Planning and Development 1982). As part of the evaluation, 4,000 questionnaires were sent to patients, supervising physicians, consulting pharmacists, coworkers, and health facility administrators. Results showed that the pharmacist-prescriber was accepted by over 95 percent of the patients and that this new role was performed competently, safely, and cost-effectively.

These favorable outcomes helped lead to the enactment of legislation. In 1983 Senate Bill 502 was passed, amending California's State Pharmacy Practice Act and permitting pharmacists practicing in "licensed health care facilities" (institutional settings such as hospitals and nursing homes) to prescribe drugs for patients under protocols established by the facility and with the authorization of the patient's physician.* It was hoped that the legislation would result in an expanded role for pharmacists and in improved prescribing in California nursing homes.

* No corresponding legislation was passed for physicians' assistants and nurse practitioners.

CHAPTER FOUR

Inappropriate Drug Use by the Elderly: The Problem of Noncompliance and Some Potential Solutions

Introduction

The frequency of inappropriate drug use by the elderly causes serious concern among experts in geriatric care. Consequences of the elderly's noncompliance with prescribed drug regimens can be disastrous:

☐ A 65-year-old patient with hypertension discontinues his medication because its side effects make him feel worse than he does when he is not on medication. His high blood pressure is no longer controlled, and he eventually has a stroke leading to prolonged hospitalization and permanent disability.

☐ An 80-year-old woman suffering from depression no longer takes her antidepressants because she sees no improvement in her condition after one week of drug therapy. She does not realize that the benefits of some antidepressants become apparent only after the drugs have been taken for several weeks.

☐ A 75-year-old patient on diuretic therapy and digoxin for congestive heart failure stops taking his potassium supplement because he finds it unpalatable. It seems to him that his condition is under control without the supplement. Eventually, he becomes hypokalemic—low in potassium. The potassium deficiency, in combination with digoxin, creates heart rhythm disturbances in the patient, which leads to an emergency room visit and subsequent hospitalization.

In this chapter we describe the kinds of problems that elderly patients encounter when taking their medications. We identify the factors associated with noncompliance, describe their particular relevance for the elderly, and discuss simple and practical strategies for preventing, detecting, and/or treating noncompliance by aged patients. We then offer a critique of existing studies examining compliance among the elderly and present an agenda for the kind of research needed in this area. The chapter concludes with a description of the staggering clinical and economic consequences of noncompliance.

Magnitude and Varieties of Noncompliance

Noncompliance is widespread among ambulatory elderly patients, especially those with chronic conditions requiring maintenance medications. The extent of noncompliance among the elderly is estimated at about 40 percent (Cooper, Love & Raffoul 1982), although a recent study has placed the estimate as high as 75 percent (Ostrom 1985).

Studies show that omission or underuse of medication is the most common form of noncompliance by elderly ambulatory patients. In one of the earliest studies investigating medication errors made by the ambulatory elderly, researchers found that 59 percent of patients made one or more errors and that 26 percent made potentially serious errors (Schwartz et al. 1962). Nearly 66 percent of the patients who made errors omitted prescribed medications. Unfortunately, the researchers did not analyze the relationship between the type of noncompliance and the type of drug being taken. Failure to take antihypertensive medications or digoxin can, for example, be far more serious than failure to take minor tranquilizers.

The prevalence of errors of omission has been discussed in other research conducted both in this nation and abroad (Lundin 1978; Wandless & Davie 1977; Hemminki & Heikkila 1975; Darnell et al. 1986). However, few studies have examined the causes of underuse. In one study investigating this problem, researchers found not only that underuse is the most prevalent type of noncompliance but also that many elderly patients who underuse prescribed drugs do so deliberately, primarily because they think that they do not need the drug in the dosage prescribed (Cooper, Love & Raffoul 1982).

Evidence corroborating this finding was obtained in a survey of psychotropic drug use among 1,101 noninstitutionalized persons aged 55 years and older (Stephens, Haney & Underwood 1982). When respondents were asked why they did not follow the directions on their prescriptions, almost half of them answered, "I don't like the medication or the prescription dosage." Almost a quarter of the responses were, "I take them [psychotropic drugs] when I feel I need them";

fewer than 10 percent answered, "I get better results taking them my own way"; and 4 percent responded, "I get bad side effects." These data suggest that a major reason why the elderly underuse medications is their dissatisfaction with some part of the drug regimen—with the type, amount, dosage schedule, and/or side effects. Because of these concerns, patients make adjustments in their drug therapy, often omitting medications to suit their perceived needs.

In order to investigate problems frequently encountered in drug use among low-income elderly living in a housing project in Seattle, J. R. Ostrom and her associates (1985) conducted home visits and carried out detailed interviews with 183 elderly persons. Although Washington state law requires that the pharmacist counsel the patient about safe and effective use of each new prescription, only 44 percent of those regularly using prescription drugs could recall that the pharmacist had instructed them on use, but 80 percent recalled that their physicians had done so. Only 52 percent reported that their physicians had informed them about possible side effects, and even fewer—30 percent—reported that their pharmacists had done so. Twenty-nine percent reported receiving only instructions for use by either physician or pharmacist, while 16 percent said that neither the physician nor the pharmacist had given them any counseling at all about the drugs prescribed.

Interviewers in the Ostrom study, by checking prescription containers and asking specific questions, identified the problems that patients encountered most frequently with prescription drugs (Table 4.1). The most frequently encountered problems regarding noncompliance were label discrepancy (discrepancies between the labeled dosage on the prescription container and the dosage actually used) and underuse of medications.

Concern about underuse of medication is based on the assumption that, like other forms of noncompliance, it is inherently undesirable. In some instances this may be true. For example, in the previously cited study conducted by Cooper and his colleagues (1982), researchers found that 50 percent of the instances of psychotropic drug noncompliance concerned the underuse of antidepressants; in other words, the subjects took the drugs only sporadically. Because antidepressants are effective only if they are taken consistently, sporadic use may interfere with the therapeutic goal.

In other cases, however, omission of medication may be beneficial. It may be a perfectly valid response by patients who want to avoid

TABLE 4.1

Frequency of Problems with Current Prescription Medications

	Frequency of occurrence	
Problem	No.	Pct.
Label discrepancy	51	37%
Underuse of medication	33	24
Cannot read label	19	14
Cannot open childproof container	17	12
Doesn't know purpose of prescription medication	9	7
Shares prescription medication with another .	9	7
Poor storage	8	6
Uses outdated prescription medication	8	6
Uses duplicate prescription	5	4
Overuse of medication	5	4

SOURCE: Adapted from Ostrom et al., *Medical Care* 23:161, February 1985.

taking an excessive number of different types of drugs or who hesitate to take large doses of a single drug (Hemminki & Heikkila 1975). This type of behavior has been called "intelligent noncompliance" (Weintraub 1976). The concept of intelligent noncompliance may be of special relevance to the elderly, for older people may omit medications in order to compensate for physiological attributes of aging or disease—attributes that affect their reactions to drugs and may be unknown to, or unrecognized by, their physicians.

The incidence, causes, and consequences of intelligent noncompliance need to be investigated because they can have adverse consequences for the health of the patient and for the physician-patient relationship. The physician, unaware of the patient's lack of compliance, may attribute changes in the patient's health to the prescribed drug therapy rather than to factors such as the course of the disease, diagnostic error, or effects of concomitant therapy. Such incorrect attributions can have serious effects. Communication between the physician and the patient is broken, and the patient's trust in the physician's judgment is undermined. Most important, the patient's recovery is hindered.

Factors Associated with Noncompliance

Although studies that address the issue of a direct association between noncompliance and aging are inconclusive, factors known to be

TABLE 4.2

Factors Associated with Noncompliance Among Geriatric Patients

Multiple drug regimens
Duration of drug treatment
Types of drugs prescribed
Chronic illness and physical and mental impairments
Social isolation
Knowledge of the drug regimen
Patient deference toward health professionals
Drug costs

associated with noncompliance are particularly characteristic of the elderly population. The factors associated with noncompliance that are particularly applicable to the elderly are listed in Table 4.2.

Multiple Drug Regimens

Studies of drug use consistently show a negative relationship between patient compliance and the number of drugs taken by the patient (Malahay 1966; Francis, Korsch & Morris 1969; Latiolais & Berry 1969; Weintraub, Au & Lasagna 1973; Hulka et al. 1975; Parkin et al. 1976; Caplan et al. 1976; Darnell et al. 1986). Taking three or more drugs increases the likelihood that the patient will be noncompliant, either deliberately or unknowingly. Because 25 percent of elderly persons consume three or more drugs as part of their daily treatment plan (compared with 9 percent of younger persons), the elderly are particularly at risk for noncompliance (American Association of Retired Persons 1984).

Duration of Drug Treatment

Studies have shown that compliance tends to decrease with time. For example, patients are more likely to take antibiotics in the first stages of treatment than in later stages (Bergman & Werner 1963; Charney et al. 1967). Other studies show that the percentage of patients who adhere carefully to treatment plans for hypertension and other chronic diseases—diseases to which the elderly are particularly susceptible—rapidly declines after the initial diagnosis and early months of treatment (Rudd et al. 1979; Haynes et al. 1982). Patients who are fully compliant during their hospitalization may become noncompliant soon after discharge (Hare & Willcox 1967; Irwin, Weitzell & Morgan 1971). The explanation for these findings might be that patients' drug therapy is closely supervised in the hospital and at initial diagnosis but is not monitored as carefully thereafter.

Types of Drugs Prescribed

Unfortunately, little research has addressed directly the relationship between compliance and types of drugs prescribed, but available studies imply that rate of compliance varies with type of drug. Compliance tends to be higher for cardiac drug regimens than for diuretics, potassium supplements, antihypertensives, and other drug classes (Closson & Kikugawa 1975; Hulka et al. 1975; Hemminki & Heikkila 1975; Spector et al. 1978; Fletcher, Pappius & Harper 1979). Evidence suggests that patients are selective, adhering to those drug regimens they consider most important to maintaining their health. Patient selectivity in compliance applies particularly to elderly patients on complex regimens. The elderly patient may be totally compliant with one part of a drug regimen and totally noncompliant with another.

Chronic Illness and Physical and Mental Impairments

The health status of the elderly—both illnesses and physical and mental impairments—makes them exceptionally vulnerable to noncompliance. Almost half of the noninstitutionalized elderly are limited in mobility because of chronic conditions. Two conditions, heart disease and arthritis, account for almost half of the activity limitation (Kovar 1977; Rice & Estes 1984). Decreased activity and dexterity can limit a person's ability and willingness to have prescriptions filled, take drugs regularly, and open and close the childproof containers that, to arthritic hands, are unmanageable.

Vision and hearing impairments, which afflict many of the elderly, also contribute to noncompliance. Eighty percent of the elderly wear glasses. Even with glasses, many have impaired vision. Failing eyesight reduces the ability to read small print on prescription labels and package inserts (Dirckx 1979). About 30 percent of the population aged 65 years and older suffer significant hearing loss (Butler & Lewis 1977; National Center for Health Statistics 1985). Yet, only 5 percent of the nation's elderly wear hearing aids. Many older people do not recognize hearing problems, are unwilling to acknowledge them, or find that hearing aids do not help. Reluctance to use hearing aids may also be related to the fact that Medicare does not reimburse beneficiaries for their cost. Hearing loss limits patients' ability to hear directions for appropriate drug use and discourages them from asking questions for fear they might not hear the answers (Ebersole & Hess 1981). Hearing loss also contributes to social isolation—another factor related to noncompliance.

To the elderly, memory loss is a critical problem. Fifteen percent of people over 60 years of age have difficulty with memory, and the percentage increases with age. For some, the problem is related to prescribed medications; for others, it is the far more serious senile dementia. Because senile dementia may be difficult to recognize in its early stages, physicians and others involved with a patient may not foresee possibilities for noncompliance.

Social Isolation

Studies have demonstrated that compliance tends to be a greater problem when patients are socially isolated (Haynes, Sackett & Taylor 1980; Hussar 1975; Blackwell 1973; Porter 1969). One study reported that medication errors were more likely to be made by elderly people living alone than by those who lived with others. Potentially serious errors were made by 42 percent of patients living alone, whereas such errors were made by 18 percent of those living with one or more persons (Schwartz et al. 1962). Social isolation is more common among the elderly, particularly among elderly women, than among people in any other age group. About 25 percent of the nation's elderly live alone, and the numbers are growing. Many have experienced not only loss of spouse but also loss of relatives, friends, and coworkers.

Knowledge of the Drug Regimen

A number of studies have observed that when a patient is provided with specific and detailed instruction about his or her particular drug regimen, compliance improves (Svarstad 1976; Hulka et al. 1976; Svarstad 1986). Researchers have found that individualized instruction (as opposed to more general directives, such as, "Take these pills as directed") is effective when the mode of communication is oral (Wilber & Barrow 1969; McKenney et al. 1973; McKenney et al.

1978; Alderman & Schoenbaum 1975; Cole & Emmanuel 1971; Mac-Donald, MacDonald & Phoenix 1977). Others have found the same results when the instruction is written (Alderman & Schoenbaum 1975; Takala et al. 1979; Gundert-Remy, Remy & Weber 1976; Gabriel, Gagnon & Bryan 1977).
A number of studies have documented that elderly people lack basic information about their drugs. They are uninformed about the name and purpose of drugs, the dosage schedules, and the duration of the regimen and its possible side effects, or adverse consequences (Schwartz et al. 1962; Cooper 1978; Lundin et al. 1980; Lofholm 1978; Klein et al. 1982). Mastery of this basic information does not ensure compliance, for, as we have seen, patients may know what they are supposed to do but refuse to do it. However, ignorance can certainly predispose patients to noncompliance.
Studies of younger patients indicate that physicians' drug instructions are given hastily at the end of the patient's visit and are usually fragmentary, incomplete, and general (Svarstad 1976, 1986). Often, patients are not given basic information, such as the purpose of the drug, expected treatment outcomes, duration of drug regimen, and dosage schedule and frequency (Hulka et al. 1976; Svarstad 1976; Francis, Korsch & Morris 1969). Sometimes patients receive no instructions at all, primarily because the physician assumes that he or she has already given instructions or that other health professionals have done so. There is no reason to believe that physician instruction of the aged is any better.

Patient Deference Toward Health Professionals

Frequently, older patients do not ask questions or express concerns to physicians or pharmacists (DeSimone, Peterson & Carlstedt 1977; Miller 1983). Their reticence has different causes. Some patients may not raise questions because of their respect for professional authority and their reluctance to challenge it. Other patients are afraid of looking unintelligent or unsophisticated. Still others are simply too sick or too anxious to ask questions.
For their part, physicians rarely invite questions or challenges from patients regarding the safety and efficacy of proposed drug therapy. When physicians do talk about a patient's regime, they often do so in ways that brook no opposition—for example, "You *are* taking all of your medications, aren't you?" Physicians may also answer questions relating to drug therapy with one- or two-word responses. Thus,

patterned deference of patients toward doctors—the conspiracy of silence—is maintained. Under these conditions, misconceptions remain uncorrected, worries remain unassuaged, and chances for noncompliance are increased. The ultimate victim, of course, is the patient, whose therapeutic outcome is compromised.

Drug Costs

Yet another barrier to compliance is economic: patients' inability to afford prescription drugs in the amounts called for by prescription directions. If elderly patients are unable to afford drugs, their health can be adversely affected. Health professionals have expressed concern particularly about the elderly who are on minimal, fixed incomes. Their inability to purchase necessary drugs may cause them to discontinue necessary drug therapy (Smith 1979; Lamy 1980; Simonson 1984). These concerns have been corroborated by elderly patients' personal accounts provided in congressional hearings.

The relationship between noncompliance and drug costs has not been the subject of much empirical research. The studies that are available, however, indicate that drug costs are a factor in noncompliance. For example, in a study of 290 chronically ill patients discharged from a general hospital in Canada, researchers found that the financial burden imposed by drug costs was the primary reason given by patients for noncompliance with drug treatment (Brand, Smith & Brand 1977). This study was unique in that researchers developed independent estimates of patients' drug expenditures to examine whether there was a relationship between drug expenditures and patients' noncompliance. Results revealed that the average monthly cost of drugs prescribed for patients who did not comply with their physicians' instructions was almost three times higher than the cost of drugs for patients who complied.

Another study of 82 chronically ill patients discharged from three acute care hospitals in Boston found that patients who were noncompliant cited the cost of drugs as a reason for their inability to follow physicians' instructions about medications (Donabedian & Rosenfeld 1964). However, researchers made no independent assessment of actual drug costs.

More recently, a study of 155 elderly residents of an urban subsidized apartment building revealed that 6.4 percent of those surveyed reported drug expenses as a problem, even though only 24 percent had insurance covering drug expenditures (Darnell et al. 1986). However, the researchers did not determine whether those who considered drug costs a problem were the individuals most likely to be noncompliant. Nor did they attempt to assess actual drug expenditures and relate these figures to compliance.

These studies are limited by small samples of elderly patients and vague definitions of compliance, which make it difficult to assess whether the subjects failed to purchase needed prescriptions because of financial constraints. However, the studies *are* important because investigators made efforts to take cost factors into account. Drug costs are often neglected in studies designed to elicit information about patients' drug therapy decisions (Testimony submitted by Helene Lipton to Senate Special Committee on Aging, U.S. Congress, July 20, 1987).

Strategies to Prevent and Treat Noncompliance Among the Elderly

To be effective in the care of patients, particularly those who have chronic illnesses and are thus prone to noncompliance, the physician must function as teacher, motivator, and persuader. As a teacher, the physician must use communication skills that ensure that the patient understands and can recall the information conveyed. To motivate the patient, the physician must use strategies designed to attract the patient's attention so that the patient listens to instructions about drug therapy. Finally, even if the patient has been motivated to listen to the physician's message and even if the message is understood and remembered, the patient will not act on it unless he or she accepts it. Therefore, the physician must also be a persuader.

Physicians who use effective communication skills have patients with higher levels of compliance than do other physicians (Svarstad 1976). Some people may argue that these kinds of skills are inborn— an inherent part of a physician's personality. However, there is compelling evidence that techniques of teaching, motivating, and persuading can be acquired. Physicians who receive training in such skills can master them and improve compliance among their patients (Inui, Yourtree & Williamson 1976).

Physician-patient communication requires that the physician have a flexible communication style, be willing to listen to the patient, and be adaptable. Svarstad (1976) found that an effective communication process involves the following:

☐ Anticipating the patient's need for information.

☐ Providing information needed by the patient.

☐ Eliciting feedback from the patient to identify communication barriers.

☐ Redesigning or tailoring the communication to meet individual patient needs.

☐ Periodically assessing the patient's motivation and knowledge in order to identify changing needs and problems.

Health professionals and researchers working with geriatric patients have proposed specific communication strategies that physicians, pharmacists, and nurses can use to improve compliance by the elderly. The purpose of these strategies is to break down the barriers to noncompliance: multiple regimen, long duration of treatment, selective compliance based on type of drug prescribed, physical and mental impairments, social isolation, lack of knowledge, patient deference toward health professionals, and drug costs.

Strategies to Deal with Multiple Drug Regimens

Physicians and pharmacists can reduce the risk of noncompliance in patients who have multiple drug regimens by placing not only the name but also the purpose of each drug on the prescription container. Labeling of this kind reduces chances for errors, especially the errors that can be made when there are prescriptions from more than one physician and/or when prescriptions are filled by many different pharmacists.

Careful labeling, of course, requires that the physician be willing to write the purpose of the drug on the prescription and that the pharmacist be willing to talk to the physician if the instructions are not clear to the patient. Such labeling should be simple, direct, and in terminology easily understood by elderly patients: for example, "digoxin—heart pill"; "ampicillin—antibiotic for infection"; and "lasix—water pill."

Another way to help patients taking multiple medications involves simplifying the regimens. Physicians and pharmacists should examine each regimen and make certain that it is the safest, simplest, and most effective therapy available. Every effort should be made to simplify scheduling. For example, instead of prescribing digoxin every other day, a physician might change the scheduling so that a smaller

TABLE 4.3

Strategies to Prevent and Treat Noncompliance Among the Elderly: Characteristics of the Drugs or Regimens

Barriers to compliance: characteristics of the drugs or regimens	Strategy
Multiple drug regimens	▪ Put name and purpose of medication on containers ▪ Label in a simple, direct, and understandable manner (e.g., "digoxin—heart pill") ▪ Simplify scheduling of medications by titrating medications against treatment response to determine the smallest amount of medication required and by eliminating unnecessary medications ▪ Use a patient profile system
Long duration of regimen	▪ Monitor for continued compliance ▪ Periodically assess patient status and review drug regimen with patient
Types of drug prescribed	▪ Put names and purposes of medication on containers ▪ Label in a simple, direct, and understandable manner

dosage is taken every day. Given the slower renal excretion rate in the older adult, this change would result in more effective therapy, as well as provide a means to improve compliance. A physician might also prescribe a medication with a long half-life on a once-daily or twice-daily basis, as opposed to three or four times daily. In addition, efforts should be made to titrate medications against treatment response in order to determine the smallest amount of medication required. Finally, whenever feasible, unnecessary medications should be eliminated (Sherman, Warach & Libow 1979). For example, the prescription of potassium supplements for a patient taking diuretics is not always necessary if the patient does not have a clinically significant potassium deficit or is not taking a digitalis preparation.

When it is not feasible or desirable to simplify a complex regimen, pharmacists may use a patient profile system to question patients about drug use and to determine whether drugs are being refilled promptly. The format of patient profiles can range from file cards to the computer-based systems that are now readily available. Prescriptions in such computer systems are filed by name as well as number. The system requirements vary, but the basic components involve a brief history of the patient to determine health status, diagnoses, current drug regimen (including both prescription and nonprescription drugs), dates of drug refills, drug allergies, health insurance coverage, and names and specialties of physicians. By maintaining patient profiles, the pharmacist can also guard against adverse reactions, drug-drug interactions that may mitigate the effects of prescription drugs, and drug-food interactions that may enhance or inhibit drug effects (see Table 4.3).

Strategies to Deal with Long Duration of Treatment and Types of Drugs Prescribed

When patients must take drugs for long periods of time and must take different types of drugs, two strategies may be helpful in assuring compliance. First, the physician or pharmacist may monitor for continued compliance by arranging for the patient to make periodic revisits and by counting pills during a visit. Second, the physician can periodically assess the patient's status and carefully review the treatment plan and specifics of treatment at each visit. Finally, the pharmacist can do a careful drug history every time the patient comes in to have a prescription filled (Table 4.3).

Strategies to Deal with Chronic Illness and Physical and Mental Impairments

As we have seen, the chronic illnesses and physical and mental impairments characteristic of old age contribute to noncompliance among the elderly. Loss of hearing, vision, memory, and dexterity are major problems affecting compliance (Table 4.4).

If a patient suffers hearing loss, the physician should determine the impact of the impairment on the patient and send the person to a specialist to determine whether the impairment is remediable. If it is not, then health professionals providing drug instructions to the hearing-impaired elderly patient should remember to speak loudly and slowly and should face the patient directly when speaking. It is also helpful to give the patient written instructions to reinforce oral directions.

Physicians may evaluate vision loss in much the same way that they evaluate hearing loss. If the impairment cannot be treated, it may be

TABLE 4.4

Strategies to Prevent and Treat Noncompliance Among the Elderly: Physical and Mental Impairments

Barriers to compliance: physical and mental impairments	Strategy
Hearing impairment that cannot be corrected	■ Speak loudly and slowly ■ Face the patient directly
Vision impairment that cannot be corrected	■ Label all written information with large letters using boldface type ■ Use a color-coding system
Memory loss	■ Distribute patient package inserts to reinforce physician, pharmacist, and nurse instructions and to serve as home reference guides[a] ■ Repeat instructions ■ Evaluate patient's comprehension of drug instructions, using nonthreatening, nonjudgmental questions ■ Use electronic bottlecap for pills
Dexterity problems	■ Advise of the availability of nonchildproof medication containers

[a] Patient package inserts (PPIs) may be especially helpful to older patients. A large prospective study of PPIs found that older patients read them more often, resulting in a small but detectable increase in patient knowledge about medications (Kanouse et al. 1981). We shall have more to say about these informational leaflets in Chapter 8.

necessary to use large letters and boldface type on written materials provided to the patient. It may be effective also to initiate a color-coding system to diminish chances for error. In such a system, a colored dot is placed on each medication container, and a dot of the same color is placed on a medication calendar at the time the medication is to be taken.

Several approaches can be used to deal with the effects of memory loss. Patient package inserts (PPIs) or similar drug information materials can be provided to elderly patients to reinforce health professionals' oral instructions and to serve as home reference guides. Another strategy involves repetition of information, which can enhance patients' ability to remember instructions about drug use. Patient comprehension of such instructions should then be evaluated through a nonthreatening, nonpatronizing line of questioning (Haynes, Sackett & Taylor 1980).

Another useful memory aid is a special bottlecap for medications. The bottlecap contains a light, an alarm, and a silicon chip, pre-programmed to specific dosing intervals. The light flashes and the alarm sounds repeatedly at predetermined dosage intervals, and both continue until the cap is removed from the bottle. Alarm volume and tones are selected for their audibility to geriatric patients, and the bottlecaps, which are not childproof, are manageable for older patients. A variety of these electronic reminder devices are currently on the market.

Loss of dexterity is another problem common among the elderly. Health professionals can reduce problems associated with limited dexterity by advising the elderly of the availability of nonchildproof medication containers (Sherman, Warach & Libow 1979).

Strategies to Deal with Social Isolation

For elderly patients living alone, physicians and pharmacists could distribute medication calendars that specify the names of medications and the times and days on which they should be taken. The usefulness of these aids in enhancing compliance has been demonstrated across age groups (Wandless & Davie 1977; Deberry, Jefferies & Light 1974; Moulding 1979). Medication calendars can be valuable reminders to older patients who have no family members or close friends to remind them when it is time to take medication. The electronic bottlecap previously suggested for patients suffering memory loss may also be useful for patients living alone (Table 4.5).

If elderly patients are living with or near relatives or close friends, every effort should be made to involve the family members or friends in strategies to improve compliance. Studies have demonstrated higher levels of compliance among patients whose families are supportive, probably because of the family's supervisory role (Haynes 1976; Shaw & Opit 1976).

Strategies to Deal with the Patient's
Lack of Knowledge

Another major impediment to compliance is the patient's lack of knowledge about safe and effective drug use. Physicians and phar-

TABLE 4.5

Strategies to Prevent and Treat Noncompliance Among the Elderly:
Social, Cognitive, Behavioral, and Economic Problems

Barriers to compliance: social, cognitive, behavioral, and economic problems	Strategy
Social isolation	▪ Distribute medication calendars ▪ Use electronic bottlecap for pills ▪ Involve available family members, friends, and others in the patient's social support network
Lack of knowledge about drug use	▪ Provide specific and detailed oral and written information about the drug regimen, including purpose and type of medication prescribed, brand or generic name, dosage schedule, duration of therapy, and information on whether the drug should be taken continuously or symptomatically
Deference toward health professionals	▪ Provide older patients time to ask questions ▪ Introduce a contingency contract
Cost of drugs	▪ Substitute generic drugs or less costly alternatives ▪ Suggest nondrug alternatives ▪ Discourage the use of unnecessary nonprescription drugs

macists, by providing elderly patients with appropriate information about their drug regimens, can play a critical role in alleviating this problem. Yet research demonstrates that specific drug information is rarely given to patients.

As we noted in Chapter 3, physicians do not spend much time with their elderly patients and spend even less time instructing them about their drugs (Svarstad 1976; Kane et al. 1980b). In addition, physicians fail to communicate in language understood by the patient and are often unaware of the patient's lack of knowledge or motivation (Korsch & Negrete 1972). Furthermore, even if the physician does communicate valuable information about drugs, the patient's anxiety and physical limitations may diminish his or her capacity to understand and remember the instructions.

It is important that health professionals deal with elderly patients' lack of knowledge by conveying certain kinds of information: purpose and/or type of medication prescribed, brand or generic name, dosage schedule, duration of therapy, and instructions on whether the drug should be taken on a continuing basis or only when symptoms arise. Investigators have found that the likelihood of compliance increases as the clinicians' instructions become more specific and individualized (Svarstad 1976; Hulka et al. 1976; McKenney et al. 1973; McKenney et al. 1978). To assure optimum results, oral instruction should be supplemented with written information.

Strategies to Deal with Patient Deference Toward Health Professionals

The problem of deference toward health professionals can be alleviated if patients are given time to ask questions. Also, if a health professional pauses at intervals and encourages a patient to respond, there is greater likelihood that the patient will participate in decisions involving the drug regimen. Still another way to involve the elderly patient actively in the decision-making process is use of the contingency contract. This agreement, usually written, allows the clinician and patient to establish a treatment goal, to specify the obligations of each party in attempting to reach that goal, and to set a time limit for its accomplishment. A large body of literature already supports the view that the provider-patient contract is a useful tool for improving patient compliance (Eraker, Kirscht & Becker 1984; Lewis & Michnich 1977; Quill 1983).

Strategies to Deal with the Problem of Drug Costs

Physicians and pharmacists can help reduce the financial burden for their elderly patients by substituting generic drugs for brand-name products, when possible, by suggesting nondrug alternatives, when feasible (e.g., dietary measures and exercise), and by discouraging the use of needless and often expensive nonprescription drugs.

A Critique of Studies on Compliance

Available studies on noncompliance in the general population are limited in several ways. One problem found in many studies is that patients' own reports are the means used to evaluate noncompliance.

It is well known that, in reporting their drug-taking behavior, patients tend to exaggerate their level of compliance. When researchers have compared use of interviews with more objective techniques, such as pill counts and laboratory tests, the findings indicate that interviews tend to show too great a degree of compliance (Gordis, Markowitz, & Lilienfeld 1969).

Research methods may also result in underestimation of the extent of unintentional noncompliance because they do not provide means of identifying patients who think that they are complying but in fact are not. In the study conducted by Stephens, Haney, and Underwood in 1982, patients were asked, "Do you always follow the prescription?" An affirmative answer was interpreted as evidence of compliant behavior. There was no way of determining whether or not patients had understood the instructions on their prescriptions. Unintentional noncompliance, then, went unidentified.

Methods used in the Cooper, Love, and Raffoul study of 1982 might also have led to underestimation of unintentional noncompliance. Interviewers asked to see patients' medication containers and then asked the patients whether each prescription drug was taken in a way that differed from the instructions on the bottle label. If the response was negative, the patient was considered compliant. To obtain evidence of compliance, interviewers might instead have asked patients how they used the drugs and then have checked instructions on their bottle labels. Similar criticism could be leveled against other studies.

Another methodological problem—one found in the study by Darnell and colleagues in 1986—is the omission of pro re nata (PRN) drugs from compliance calculations. PRN drugs are to be taken only "as needed," but many patients do not understand the directions and take such drugs on a scheduled basis. Obviously, failure to include these drugs could lead to underestimation of the magnitude of patients' noncompliance.

Even though factors associated with noncompliance are especially prevalent among the elderly, there has been little systematic theoretical and empirical research done to compare compliance and medication-taking behavior among older persons with compliance and medication-taking behavior among younger persons. Most drug research has, in fact, been conducted on young people who are in relatively good health (Wynne & Heller 1973). Some studies conclude that noncompliance, known to be widespread among the elderly, is more prevalent among the aged than among other groups. Other studies suggest that advancing age is associated with increased compliance. A comprehensive review of available research on compliance concludes that most studies indicate no relationship between age and compliance (Sackett & Haynes 1976).

Those few researchers who have studied this relationship have not examined other variables simultaneously. They could not, therefore, discover how the age-compliance relationship may be affected when additional variables are present. For example, the elderly may be more likely to be noncompliant only when certain risk factors are present (e.g., when they are on complex regimen, when they live alone, or when the physician fails to provide adequate information). These kinds of interaction effects cannot be identified unless patient age, as a variable, is examined simultaneously with other variables, such as nature of drug regimen, living arrangements, and physician-patient relationship. It is necessary, therefore, for researchers to use multivariate techniques to shed light on the problem.

In many drug studies researchers have failed to address adequately the multiple factors that may be responsible for compliance or noncompliance, because they have measured single rather than multiple outcomes. Compliance is determined by patient motivation as well as by patient knowledge. It may be possible, then, that the elderly, because of worries about health, have an increased motivation to comply but have, because of decreased memory capacity, a diminished ability to retain long and complex instructions. These effects, called suppressor effects, act in opposite ways and could cancel each other out. As a result, a study might find no relationship between age and compliance. On the other hand, if one effect were stronger in an individual, or cumulatively, in a study group, a positive or negative effect might be seen. However, the explanation of these apparently inconsistent results would be found only by properly dividing up the relation of age and compliance into a set of effects which work in different directions.

Another problem with many studies relates to the way in which individuals are selected to participate in the research. Studies often exclude subjects who are regarded as unreliable or too difficult to locate and interview, such as patients with dementia or aphasia or those with hearing difficulties (Klein et al. 1982; Spector et al. 1978; Davis 1968). Because more elderly people than younger people would fit these categories and thus be excluded, the elderly who are most vulnerable to noncompliance may not have been participants in many studies. The studies may, then, inaccurately show a lower rate of noncompliance than actually exists among the aged.

Although research is inconclusive about whether or not elderly patients are more compliant than are younger patients, in absolute terms the number of elderly patients using prescription drugs inappropriately is substantial. As we have shown, factors known to be associated with noncompliance are prevalent among the elderly population, making them especially at risk for noncompliance. Clinicians, however, should not interpret these factors as evidence that elderly patients are not complying with therapy. Health professionals should, instead, use them as guidelines to identify patients for whom noncompliance could be a problem and for whom intervention strategies might be appropriate.

Drug Compliance by the Elderly: A Research Agenda

There is need for research in specific areas related to compliance among the elderly. As noted earlier, failure to take medication constitutes a major kind of noncompliance among the aged. Some researchers have argued that the elderly's failure to take as many drugs as prescribed is deliberate (Weintraub 1976). Other researchers contend that failure to take medication is unintentional (Lundin 1980; Hulka et al. 1976). Perhaps both intentional and unintentional noncompliance occur for different types of drugs and among different segments of the aged. Sophisticated studies of the "error by omission" phenomenon would help clarify the problem and point the way to its resolution.

As previously discussed, certain factors predispose people of any age to noncompliance. However, no investigators have tried to determine the underlying reasons for this predisposition. Why, for example, are patients who take multiple drugs more vulnerable to problems of noncompliance than are other patients? Does an informational problem exist? Do patients on such regimens fail to receive, or to hear, adequate information regarding their medications, and do their subsequent ignorance, confusion, and misconceptions result in greater numbers of drug errors? Or is the problem a motivational one? Are patients who take several drugs simultaneously likely to experience side effects, thus reducing their willingness to comply? Or is there a life-style problem? Do patients on a long-term or multiple drug regimen consider such a regimen disruptive and inconvenient, and thus tend to comply less readily? Or does noncompliance involve some combination of all of these factors? Future research efforts should focus on the reasons for the inverse relationship between complexity of drug regimen and compliance, so that clinicians may develop effective intervention strategies.

Similarly, the reasons for the correlation between social isolation and noncompliance require further exploration. Are those living alone more likely to forget to take their medications simply because they do not have people to remind them? Or are they less motivated to comply because feelings of depression and loneliness reduce their desire to take their drugs as directed? As the number of elderly persons living alone continues to grow, the need to explore this relationship becomes compelling.

Numerous studies have reported that the elderly lack basic information about both prescribed and nonprescribed drugs, but the underlying cause for this is uncertain. Do physicians fail to give adequate information to their elderly patients? Or do such patients fail to hear or understand physicians' instructions? Researchers have found that patients presented with standardized drug instructions show wide variation in their ability to interpret the instructions correctly (Mazulla, Lasagna & Griner 1974). Are elderly patients reluctant to pose drug-related questions and problems to health providers? A survey of pharmacist-patient interaction suggests that this is so (DeSimone, Peterson & Carlstedt 1977). So, too, does a recent FDA study, which found that only 2 percent of patients in the sample asked their physicians about their medications (Miller 1983). Do other problems exist in physician-patient and pharmacist-patient communication? Few empirical studies have explored the communication that takes place between health professionals and their elderly patients. Yet, evidence suggests that the elderly are aware of their lack of drug information and want more information about their medications (Lundin 1978; Plant 1977; American Association of Retired Persons 1984).

There are no systematic studies of the techniques that physicians use to educate and motivate their elderly patients with regard to drug therapy. Such research might answer some perplexing questions. For example, why are compliance rates for those who use cardiac drugs (e.g., digoxin) higher than the rates for those who use drugs from other classes (e.g., psychotropic medications, antihypertensives)? Do physicians spend more time instructing patients about the use of cardiac drugs because of potential adverse effects? Do they devote more energy to motivating and persuading their patients to take such drugs and more time emphasizing their importance and efficacy? Do physicians monitor use of such drugs more carefully?

Studies of physician-patient interaction could pinpoint the reasons for variability in compliance rates and the specific communication techniques that could be used to enhance elderly patients' safe and effective use of specific classes of drugs. Studies of this kind could, for example, increase understanding of psychotropic drug use among the aged in ambulatory settings. To what extent is use of these drugs initiated by elderly patients themselves? To what extent do physicians suggest nondrug alternatives? It is important to determine what proportion of the elderly's visits to physicians are caused by social problems and by need for support rather than by strictly medical problems. There should also be an assessment of the extent to which the elderly are attempting to resolve psychosocial problems by taking mood-altering medications rather than by seeking social supports in the community.

Consequences of Noncompliance

Adoption of the proposed research agenda becomes more compelling when the consequences of noncompliance are considered. Medical side effects are only one consequence of inappropriate drug use by the elderly. The economic consequences are enormous, for noncompliance can result in the need for medical services, particularly in hospitalization. Some researchers suggest that about 10 percent of hospital admissions result from poor patient compliance and that geriatric patients are particularly at risk (Graham & Livesley 1983; Frisk, Cooper & Campbell 1977).

Noncompliance, of course, is not the only cause of drug-related hospitalizations. As we have already mentioned, adverse drug reactions—often resulting from inappropriate physician prescribing—are also implicated. There is evidence to suggest that patient noncompliance and adverse drug reactions taken together account for about 15 percent of geriatric hospitalizations (McKenney & Harrison

1976; Bergman & Wiholm 1981; Livesley 1983; Frisk, Cooper & Campbell 1977; Williamson 1979; Caranasos, Stewart & Cluff 1974). The costs of such illnesses are significant. The estimated annual cost of drug-related hospital admissions of the elderly, along with their subsequent treatment, was $4.5 billion in 1983 (Pennsylvania Blue Shield 1985). However, the other costs of noncompliance—impaired quality of life, compromised health status, and needless death—can never be fully calculated.

Drug Economics and Regulation

CHAPTER FIVE

Drug Costs and the Elderly

Introduction

The following is an extract from testimony submitted by a senior citizen before the U.S. House of Representatives, Subcommittee on Health and the Environment, at a hearing on "Prescription Drug Price Increases" (July 15, 1985).

I have to take it [this medicine] every day. My doctor says I will have to take it as long as I live. . . . Medicare doesn't pay it, they said. . . . But it is hard on us. It is very hard. We don't have no other kind of income, and medicine, this medicine when I first started to get it, this Theo-Dur was $8 something, now it will run you $17 something. . . . These pain pills are $28.49, and I have to take them three times a day. It is just rough on you when you don't have no other income [but Social Security] . . . and I have to get this refilled sometimes twice a month, the arthritis pills, so I will be able to walk. . . . [The] little food I buy, then I have insurance to pay, my health insurance, my fire insurance, all that to pay, my telephone bill, my gas bill, all of that comes out of that one little check, and it is rough.

The cost of prescription drugs has long posed problems for millions of elderly who are chronically ill. After the enactment of Medicare, drugs became one of the largest out-of-pocket medical care expenditures for aged persons. In 1967, at President Johnson's direction, the Task Force on Prescription Drugs was established as part of the U.S. Department of Health, Education, and Welfare. After it had done a comprehensive study of the problems involved in extending Medicare to cover the cost of prescription drugs, the Task Force recommended that Medicare include an outpatient drug insurance program. Although many bills were introduced in Congress to achieve this goal in the late 1960s and early 1970s, such legislation was never passed. There is now renewed congressional interest in the issue of outpatient prescription drug coverage for Medicare beneficiaries, especially for those who incur "catastrophic" drug charges. In the summer of 1987 the House of Representatives passed a bill that would cover prescription drug costs for elderly Medicare beneficiaries whose drug charges exceeded $500 per year.

Although many of the private health insurance policies that are purchased by elderly individuals to supplement Medicare include some coverage for drugs, few provide full prescription drug coverage. As a result, drug costs, totaling $2.3 billion for the noninstitutionalized aged in 1980, are a significant problem for millions of elderly. Although aged Medicare beneficiaries made up only 10.9 percent of the noninstitutionalized population in 1980, their prescription drug use and drug expenditures corresponded to a disproportionate 28.6 percent of national prescription drug use and 30.2 percent of national drug expenditures (LaVange & Silverman 1987). This pattern of drug expenditures parallels personal health care expenditures. Although the aged accounted for 31 percent of expenditures for personal health care in 1980, they represented only 11 percent of the population (Hodgson & Kopstein 1984).

Surveys of the elderly have consistently shown that they want Medicare to provide outpatient drug coverage. This chapter examines the issue of prescription drug costs for the elderly and describes some mechanisms through which older people's drug costs could be controlled and, thus, their financial burden reduced.

National Health Care Expenditures for Drugs

According to figures reported by the Health Care Financing Administration (HCFA), national expenditures for "drugs and medical sundries"—a category that includes prescription and nonprescription drugs and medical sundries dispensed through retail channels—accounted for 6.7 percent of health spending, or $30.6 billion, in 1986 (Office of National Cost Estimates 1987). Approximately 56 percent of the "drugs and medical sundries" expenditures are for prescription drugs, 29 percent for nonprescription drugs, and 15 percent for other medical sundries.* Estimates of national expenditures are

*The source of the data for drugs and medical sundries is the estimate of personal consumption expenditures compiled by the Department of Commerce as part of the national income accounts. This methodology is described in detail at the end of the annual articles on national health care expenditures published by HCFA (Levit et al. 1985).

compiled annually by type of service (i.e., hospital care, physicians' services, nursing home care, drugs and medical sundries, etc.) and by source of funds (government or private). The types of services for which estimates are produced and the dollar estimates for the year 1986 are shown in Table 5.1. Expenditures for "drugs and medical sundries" include only those items purchased by consumers in retail outlets. To avoid duplicate counting, the government excludes from this category drugs provided to hospital inpatients and outpatients and to patients in nursing homes, as well as drugs dispensed directly by physicians. The latter expenditures are included under the categories of "hospital care," "nursing home care," and "physicians' services."

The exclusions from the "drugs and medical sundries" category are particularly relevant to the elderly, whose per capita rate of hospitalization and institutionalization in nursing homes exceeds that of any other age group (Waldo & Lazenby 1984). For example, the total number of hospital care days per year for aged patients is over four times that of other patients. Over one-fourth of all people discharged from community hospitals in 1980 were elderly, and this group accounted for over one-third of the days. Although those 75 years of age or older represented 4 percent of the population in 1980, they accounted for more than 20 percent of the days spent in community hospitals (Kovar 1983).

It would be valuable for the government to report how much of the expenditures included in categories other than "drugs and medical sundries" are drug expenditures. Such information would give us an estimate of total national expenditures for drugs. We can see, however, that the "drugs and medical sundries" category represents an underestimate of total drug expenditures, especially as these expenditures relate to the elderly.

The most careful, thorough, and painstaking study to date of total expenditures for drugs in the United States was one conducted by le Centre de Recherche pour l'Étude et l'Observation des Conditions de Vie (CREDOC), based in France (Glarmet-Lenoir & Hérisson 1980). In this study hospital charges for prescription drugs were estimated to be $5.5 billion in 1978.* Of the $5.5 billion, $1.5 billion was spent

*According to data from the U.S. Department of Commerce, Interindustry Division, if hospital acquisition costs for drugs, rather than hospital charges, had been used to estimate hospital expenditures for drugs, the estimate would be approximately 45 percent lower (U.S. Department of Commerce, Bureau of Economic Analysis 1984).

TABLE 5.1

National Health Expenditures by Type of Expenditure and Sources of Funds, 1986
(billions of dollars)

Expenditure category	Total all sources	Private				Government		
		Total	Consumer			Total	Federal	State and local
			Total	Out of pocket	Private insurance	Other			
National health expenditures	$458.2	$268.5	$256.9	$116.1	$140.7	$11.7	$189.7	$134.7	$55.0
Health services and supplies	442.0	262.5	256.9	116.1	140.7	5.6	179.5	126.6	52.9
Personal health care	404.0	244.1	239.0	116.1	122.9	5.0	160.0	121.8	38.1
Hospital care	179.6	83.9	81.7	16.8	64.9	2.2	95.7	76.5	19.2
Physician services	92.0	64.9	64.8	26.2	38.7	0.1	27.1	22.0	5.0
Dentist services	29.6	29.0	29.0	19.1	9.9	—	0.6	0.3	0.3
Other professional services	14.1	10.0	9.9	6.2	3.7	0.1	4.0	3.0	1.0
Drugs and medical sundries	30.6	27.3	27.3	22.9	4.5	—	3.2	1.7	1.5
Eyeglasses and appliances	8.2	6.5	6.5	5.5	1.0	—	1.7	1.6	0.2
Nursing home care	38.1	20.0	19.8	19.4	0.3	0.3	18.1	10.1	8.0
Other personal health care	11.9	2.4	—	—	—	2.4	9.5	6.5	3.0
Program administration and net cost of health insurance	24.5	18.4	17.8	—	17.8	0.6	6.1	3.4	2.7
Government public health activity	13.4	—	—	—	—	—	13.4	1.4	12.0
Research and construction	16.3	6.0	—	—	—	6.0	10.2	8.0	2.2
Research	8.2	0.4	—	—	—	0.4	7.8	7.2	0.7
Construction	8.0	5.6	—	—	—	5.6	2.4	0.9	1.5

SOURCE: Health Care Financing Administration, Office of the Actuary, Division of National Cost Estimates.

NOTES: Research and development expenditures of drug companies and other manufacturers and providers of medical equipment and supplies are excluded from noncommercial research, being implicitly included in the value of the good or service being produced. "Other Private Funds" include spending by philanthropy, industrial inplant health services, and privately financed construction.

for outpatient, and $4.0 billion for inpatient prescription drugs. The CREDOC study does not contain an estimate of hospital expenditures for nonprescription drugs and medical sundries. Thus, total hospital expenditure for drugs and medical sundries in 1978 probably exceeded $5.5 billion, although it is difficult to say by how much. This $5.5 billion expenditure for drugs dispensed to hospital inpatients and outpatients is over one-third of the $15.1 billion total expenditure for drugs and medical sundries dispensed through retail channels estimated by HCFA for that year, and it is more than 60 percent of the $8.4 billion expenditure for prescription drugs dispensed only through retail channels (Scitovsky 1982).

The CREDOC study also estimates expenditures for prescription drugs dispensed in nursing homes (just over $490 million in 1978) and for those purchased by patients from physicians ($730 million in 1978). The CREDOC estimate of expenditures for prescription drugs dispensed through retail outlets was $10.4 billion, almost $2.0 billion above the HCFA estimate for that year, whereas the study's estimate of expenditures for nonprescription drugs was almost $1.2 billion below the HCFA estimate. The total expenditures for prescription drugs, nonprescription drugs, and medical sundries in the United States in 1978 was estimated by CREDOC to be $22.5 billion. This is almost 50 percent more than the HCFA estimate, which, following national income accounting conventions that are used to avoid duplicate counting, places drug costs incurred through hospitals, nursing homes, and physician dispensing in other categories (Table 5.2). If the relationship found by CREDOC in 1978 remains constant from year to year, it translates into a national drug expenditure in the United States of approximately $46 billion in 1986.

Consumer Expenditures for Prescription Drugs

In discussing prescription drug costs, it is important to note the proportion of costs borne directly by consumers. In 1986, direct payments by patients for all personal health care amounted to $116.1 billion (29 percent of total personal health care expenditures), or about $465 per person (Office of National Cost Estimates 1987). The share of expenditures borne by the consumer varies by type of service and is higher for drugs and medical sundries dispensed through retail channels than for any other major health service. Consumers bear 9 percent of hospital costs, 29 percent of the cost of physicians' services, 51 percent of the cost of nursing home services, 64 percent

TABLE 5.2

Expenditures for Drugs and Medical Sundries,
HCFA and CREDOC Estimates, 1978

(millions of dollars)

Type of expenditure	HCFA estimates	CREDOC estimates
Consumer expenditures of pre-scription drugs in retail outlets	$ 8,455	$10,419
Consumer expenditures of non-prescription drugs and medical sundries in retail outlets	6,643	5,279
Subtotal, retail outlets	$15,098	$15,968
Prescription drugs dispensed in:		
Hospitals	—	5,535
Nursing homes	—	491
Physicians' offices	—	730
Subtotal, other than retail outlets	—	$ 6,756
Grand Total	—[a]	$22,454

SOURCE: Adapted from Scitovsky 1982:473.

[a] HCFA does not publish an estimate of total spending for drugs because prescription drugs dispensed in hospitals, nursing homes, and physicians' offices are included under the larger categories of "hospital care," "nursing home care," and "physicians' services," and drug expenditures are not analyzed separately.

of the cost of dental services, and 75 percent of the cost of drugs and medical sundries purchased through retail outlets.

Drugs dispensed through retail outlets represent one of the largest out-of-pocket medical expenses for all age groups, including the elderly. In 1986, direct out-of-pocket expenditures for drugs dispensed through retail outlets amounted to $22.9 billion, exceeded only by the $26.2 billion spent directly for physicians' services (Table 5.1).

Table 5.3 shows that the percentage of annual expenses for prescribed medicines dispensed through retail channels and paid out-of-pocket by the family was about 73 percent for the entire population in 1977. This share was slightly higher for persons 65 years or older (77 percent) than for younger persons (70.6 to 73.6 percent). The share of annual expenses for prescribed medicines paid by private insurance was 13.6 percent for the entire population and 10.3 percent for the elderly. The share of annual prescription drug expenses paid by Medicaid was 7.7 percent for the total population and 9.5 percent for the elderly. These figures are fairly consistent with results from a 1980 survey indicating that approximately 68 percent of total charges incurred by aged Medicare beneficiaries for prescription drugs were paid out-of-pocket; 13.9 percent were paid by private insurance; and 10.8 percent were paid by Medicaid (LaVange & Silverman 1987).

Medicaid Expenditures for Prescription Drugs

Medicaid is a program for the poor, funded jointly by the federal and state governments. It is a means-tested program: only those whose incomes and assets fall below certain government-determined levels are eligible for benefits. Under Medicaid, states must provide coverage for several basic services, including inpatient and outpatient hospital care, physicians' treatment, laboratory and x-ray work, and nursing home and home health services. States also have the option of covering a variety of other goods and services, including costs of prescription drugs provided outside of hospitals and nursing homes. In fact, all states, except Alaska and Wyoming, cover prescription drugs dispensed through retail outlets as an option under Medicaid.

Of the 22.1 million Medicaid recipients in the country in 1981, approximately 3.5 million (15.8 percent) were elderly (unpublished Medicaid statistics, 1981).* In contrast to Medicare, Medicaid has been a major source of payment for prescription drugs for the elderly. In 1981 the cost of drugs amounted to $609 million, 6.1 percent of all Medicaid spending for the elderly. In that year almost 80 percent of older enrollees used the prescription drug benefit (U.S. Department of Health and Human Services, Health Care Financing Administration 1983).

Throughout the 1980s, many states imposed limits on drug coverage for Medicaid beneficiaries. For example, nineteen states have co-payments on prescriptions ranging from about $.50 to $3.00. Eleven states limit the number of prescriptions that Medicaid will fill for a given patient per month, with the maximum often set as low as three prescriptions. Twenty-eight states limit the number of refills allowed per month. Partly as a result of such policies, the annual rate of increase in Medicaid expenditures for prescription drugs declined from 14.5 percent in the years before 1981 to 8.2 percent in the years after. The decline reflects both a small decrease in the number of Medicaid recipients and a 2 percent drop in real services per recipient (Holahan & Cohen 1986).

---

*The estimate of the number of elderly may be slightly low, because some elderly beneficiaries receiving benefits under the "blind" or "disabled" categories are not included in the "aged" category.

TABLE 5.3

Annual Expenditures and Sources of Payment for Prescribed Medicines Dispensed Through Retail Channels: Mean Expense Per Person with Expense and Percent Paid by Source of Payment

Age in years	Total population with expense for prescribed medicines (in 1,000s)	Mean expense per person with expense	Source of payment (pct. distribution)			
			Family	Private health insurance	Medicaid	Other[a]
Less than 6	11,736	$20	73.6%	10.2%	9.9%	6.2%
6 to 18	21,905	20	74.7	12.2	7.6	5.5
19 to 24	11,424	27	71.4	11.8	9.6	7.2
25 to 54	45,062	44	70.6	15.8	6.0	7.5
55 to 64	13,720	79	71.5	16.2	7.0	5.3
65 or older	16,577	93	77.0	10.3	9.5	3.2
Total	120,424	$46	73.0%	13.6%	7.7%	5.6%

SOURCE: Kasper 1982; NMCES household data from United States 1977.

[a] Includes CHAMPUS, CHAMPVA, the Indian Health Service, the Veterans Administration, the military, other federal, state, city, or county payers, philanthropic institutions, and unknown sources of payment.

These efforts at cost-containment may boomerang. Restrictions imposed on reimbursement for drugs may deprive elderly people of access to essential drugs. For example, in one state that limited Medicaid reimbursement for drugs to three prescriptions per month, chronically ill Medicaid recipients decreased significantly their use of several life-saving drugs, including insulin, digoxin, and certain antihypertensive agents (Soumerai et al. 1987). Patients who cannot afford to take needed drugs may develop serious complications requiring hospital care.

Per Capita Prescription Drug Use and Costs for the Elderly

A national household survey sponsored by the National Center for Health Services Research (NCHSR) in 1977 found that, of the approximately 120 million noninstitutionalized persons who took drugs, each person received an average of 7.5 prescriptions.* The number of prescriptions received by persons using drugs varied markedly with age: children under 6 years received an average of 4 prescriptions each year, whereas people 65 years of age and over received an average of 14 prescriptions (Kasper 1982).

The relationship between number of drugs prescribed and age was further established in a study conducted in 1980, called the National Medical Care Utilization and Expenditure Survey (NMCUES). This national household survey of the noninstitutionalized population found that the number of prescription drugs used increased with age. Beneficiaries 65 to 69 years of age received an average of 10 prescriptions per year, whereas those 70 to 74 years received 12 prescriptions, and those 75 to 79 received 15 prescriptions. This trend, however, did not continue for those aged 80 and over, probably because of the high rate of institutionalization in this group (LaVange & Silverman 1987).

More recent estimates derived from the National Prescription Audit[†] suggest much the same pattern. In 1982 people from 45 to 54 years of age received an average of approximately 6.9 prescriptions per

*This survey was called the National Medical Care Expenditure Survey (NMCES), and its results were not published until 1982. No data are available yet from a similar survey conducted in 1987.

[†]The National Prescription Audit (NPA) is based on data from approximately 1,200 pharmacies having computerized drug information systems. The NPA provides national estimates of the number of prescriptions dispensed from retail pharmacies.

TABLE 5.4

Out-of-Pocket Expenses for Prescribed Medicines: Percent Distribution of Persons with and without Prescribed Medicines, by Intervals of Out-of-Pocket Expense

Age in years	Total population (in 1,000s)	Out-of-pocket expense (pct. distribution)						No prescribed medicine
		None	$1 to $49	$50 to $99	$100 to $249	$250 or more		
Less than 6	18,216	10.6%	51.0%	3.4%	0.4%[a]	0.0%		34.5%
6 to 18	50,647	7.7	34.7	1.6	0.5	0.0		55.4
19 to 24	22,299	8.9	40.1	3.2	0.8	0.1[a]		46.8
25 to 54	78,472	7.9	41.7	5.8	3.2	0.5		40.9
55 to 64	20,180	6.9	40.5	10.2	9.3	2.2		30.9
65 or older	22,284	6.6	34.7	14.8	15.7	3.3		24.8
Total	212,098	8.0%	39.8%	5.7%	3.9%	0.8%		41.8%

SOURCES: Kasper 1982; NMCES household data from United States 1977.

NOTE: 0.0 indicates quantity greater than 0.00 but less than 0.05.

[a] Relative standard error is equal to or greater than 30 percent.

person; people aged 55 to 64 received about 9.3; people 65 to 74 received about 13.6; and people 75 and older averaged about 16.9 prescriptions (Baum, Kennedy & Forbes 1985). These figures may underestimate total drug use because they include prescriptions dispensed only through retail pharmacies, not through such outlets as discount houses and mail-order pharmacies. Furthermore, the figures of prescription drug use take into account only prescription drug use by outpatients, which accounts for only about half of the total drug use by the elderly. The elderly are obviously more likely to receive drugs as inpatients than are people in other age groups, because older people are more often hospitalized or placed in nursing homes.

Not only does the average number of drugs prescribed increase with age but so does the average price of prescriptions (Fisher 1980; Kasper 1982; Trapnell 1979). The relationship between age and average price per prescription is explored in detail in the Appendixes, where we also analyze factors accounting for growth in average charge per prescription for the total population. Nevertheless, it is important to note here that the average price per prescription for the elderly increased steadily from $4.00 in 1967 to $8.05 in 1980, a 101 percent increase (LaVange & Silverman 1987). Recent estimates from the Office of the Actuary, Health Care Financing Administration, give the average cost per prescription per aged beneficiary as approximately $16 in 1986 and $17 in 1987 (Waldo 1987). The 101 percent increase between 1967 and 1980 was probably caused by factors such as the introduction of expensive new drugs into the marketplace, the continuing trend toward increasing prescription size (e.g., average prescription size for drugs used by the elderly rose 22 percent from 1967 to 1973), and drug price inflation.

Because they use more drugs and pay higher prices for prescriptions than do people in other age groups, the elderly are more likely to incur large drug costs. According to the 1977 NCHSR study, 75.2 percent of the elderly obtained prescription medicines dispensed through pharmacies or other retail outlets, compared with 58.2 percent of the population as a whole. These figures are reflected in drug expenditures by the elderly. In 1977 the drug expense for persons taking at least one prescription drug averaged $46 per person for the total population but $93 per person for those 65 years of age and older. More detailed analyses revealed that 19 percent of the nation's elderly incurred annual prescription drug expenditures of $100 or more in 1977, compared with 4.7 percent of the population as a whole. These data are extremely important because they are the first precise figures available for out-of-pocket expenses for prescribed medicine analyzed by increments of increasing out-of-pocket expense for the entire non-institutionalized population (see Table 5.4).

The conclusion that persons 65 years or older use more prescription drugs, incur greater prescription drug expenses, and pay higher out-of-pocket drug expenses than the general population is consistent with the results of the NMCUES survey conducted in 1980. The NMCUES survey reported that the average number of prescriptions (12.1) and the average annual charges ($98) for aged Medicare beneficiaries were about three times greater than those for both the general population (4.6 prescriptions and $35) and for people under 65 years of age (3.7 prescriptions and $27). In fact, researchers in this survey found that one out of five aged Medicare beneficiaries spent over $160 for prescription drugs in 1980 (LaVange & Silverman 1987).

The most recent estimates of drug utilization and drug expenditures by the elderly have been provided by Daniel Waldo of the Health Care Financing Administration (Waldo 1987). His study is important not only because it integrates information from several national surveys but also because it includes the institutionalized elderly and forecasts drug use and expenditures through 1991. Waldo estimates the average number of prescriptions for aged Medicare beneficiaries at 17.1 in 1986, 17.4 in 1987, and 17.7 in 1988. Average prescription drug expenditures for aged Medicare enrollees will be $336 in 1988; this figure is projected to be $424 by 1991, a 26 percent increase. Further, Waldo projects that 31 percent of all Medicare beneficiaries (a category including the disabled) will incur total outpatient drug expenditures of $500 or more in 1988; by 1991, the corresponding figure will be 39 percent. (This $500 figure is the amount targeted in the House bill passed in 1987 as constituting "catastrophic" drug costs.)

The Impact of Rising Drug Prices on the Elderly

To appreciate fully the impact of high out-of-pocket drug expenditures on older people, it is necessary to examine the elderly's current economic status. First, however, it is important to acknowledge that since the 1960s a great deal of progress has been made toward reducing the number of elderly living below the poverty level. In 1970 almost 25 percent of persons aged 65 years and over were living below the poverty level. Five years later, the proportion had fallen to approximately 14 percent and has remained relatively stable since. In 1983, 3.7 million elderly persons were living in poverty. It should be kept in mind, however, that the official poverty index in that year was $4,775 yearly per person 65 years of age and over, which represents a low estimate of living needs. In 1983 the median annual income for elderly men was $9,766; the comparable figure for elderly women was $5,599 (Leadership Council of Aging Organizations 1983). In that same year, the median elderly household income level was $11,718, whereas the median household income of the nonelderly population was $23,865 (American Association of Retired Persons 1985). This trend has been consistent for the past several years.

There are additional reasons for concern. The poverty rate for those aged 65 years and over continues to be high, compared with the rate for other age groups. In fact, it is exceeded only by the poverty rate for persons under 25 years of age (U.S. Bureau of the Census 1984). Poverty figures, moreover, do not reveal that there are many older Americans whose income levels are just above the poverty threshold. An estimated 8.3 percent of those 65 years and over—2.2 million persons—were estimated to fall into the "near-poor" category in 1983 (i.e., subsisting on an income just above the poverty threshold). Such persons are particularly vulnerable to, and burdened by, out-of-pocket drug expenditures because, generally, they are not eligible for Medicaid.

The harsh economic realities are compounded for elderly single women and minorities (McNeely 1983; Fuller & Martin 1980). Thirty-eight percent of aged blacks and 31 percent of aged Hispanics live at extreme poverty levels (U.S. House Select Committee on Aging 1981). Approximately one half of all the aged poor are widows or single women who live alone (U.S. House Select Committee on Aging 1978; Estes, Gerard & Clarke 1984). This group is most likely to incur out-of-pocket drug expenditures that are beyond their means because of their diminished finances and their increased incidence of health problems, which create a need for prescription drugs. Although women living below the poverty line generally have access to health care through Medicaid, the many other women who are "near-poor" or on "moderate" incomes do not have the financial means to obtain adequate insurance to cover health service costs, including the cost of prescription drugs.

TABLE 5.5

Percent Distribution for Payments for Prescription Drugs Used by Poor, Near-Poor, and
Nonpoor Noninstitutionalized, Aged Medicare Beneficiaries: United States, 1980

Poverty level	Total	Source of payment (pct. distribution)				
		Medicare	Medicaid	Private plans	Out-of-pocket	Other	Unknown source or unpaid amount
Poor	100.0%	3.0%	28.4%	7.7%	58.7%	a	0.5%
Near-poor	100.0	2.7	8.3	10.7	74.1	3.9	0.2
Nonpoor	100.0	3.6	3.8	20.6	67.4	4.1	0.5
Total	100.0%	3.1%	10.8%	13.9%	68.2%	3.6%	0.4%

SOURCE: NMCUES (LaVange & Silverman 1987).

NOTE: Categorization of poor, near-poor, and nonpoor beneficiaries is based on annual family income relative to the 1980 U.S. Bureau of the Census definition of poverty level.

a Relative standard error is greater than 50 percent, or sample size is less than 20.

These income and poverty statistics provide a background for examining the elderly's out-of-pocket health care costs. The elderly's per capita out-of-pocket expenses for health care services in 1984 were estimated to be $1,000; these estimates exclude premium payments for Medicare Part B* and premiums for other health insurance policies purchased by Medicare beneficiaries (Waldo & Lazenby 1984). When such payments are included, estimates for the elderly's out-of-pocket health care expenditures total $1,500 per capita (U.S. House Select Committee on Aging 1984). Information on out-of-pocket drug costs for the elderly, broken out by economic status, was obtained in the 1980 NMCUES survey.† Results of this study revealed that the proportion of prescription drug expenses reimbursed by private insurance was similar among poor and near-poor elderly (7.7 percent and 10.7 percent, respectively) and significantly higher among those who were not poor (20.6 percent). Those elderly people whose income was just above the poverty level were least likely to have coverage for prescription drug charges; almost 75 percent of their drug expenses were paid for out-of-pocket (see Table 5.5).

Although all three groups, including those living below the poverty level, had to pay over half of their drug expenses out-of-pocket, it is clear that the near-poor are particularly vulnerable to the burden of out-of-pocket drug costs. However, the elderly poor incurred higher average annual drug expenses, and higher out-of-pocket drug expenses as a percent of family income, than did the near-poor and non-poor. In fact, the financial burden of out-of-pocket drug expenses was six times greater for the poor elderly than for those elderly who were not poor (LaVange & Silverman 1987).

It is important to note that this information was collected in 1980, before the escalation of drug prices (to be discussed in the next sec-

*Medicare Part A covers inpatient hospital services, skilled nursing facility services, home health agency services, and hospice care. Medicare Part B includes the services of physicians and other health care providers (e.g., physical and occupational therapists) and outpatient hospital services (e.g., laboratory and x-ray services).

†The sample in NMCUES was classified into three groups, based on reported 1980 family income relative to the 1980 poverty level, as defined by the Bureau of the Census: (1) poor, (2) near-poor, and (3) nonpoor. The "poor" were those Medicare beneficiaries living in families whose income level was less than or equal to the poverty level. (In 1980 the poverty level was approximately $8,000 for a family of four.) The "near-poor" were those in families whose income was above the poverty level but less than or equal to twice the poverty level, while the "nonpoor" were those in families whose income was greater than twice the poverty level (LaVange & Silverman 1987).

tion). The poor and near-poor elderly's incomes have remained relatively static in recent years (their Social Security payments have increased at about the same rate as general inflation), but their expenditures for drugs have increased dramatically because of drug price inflation. Therefore, their out-of-pocket drug expenditures relative to income are probably even greater now than they were at the time of the 1980 survey.

National surveys conducted by the American Association of Retired Persons (AARP) in 1985 and 1986 provide additional insights into the elderly's burden of out-of-pocket drug costs. Survey results revealed that over half of those aged 65 and older who were taking prescription drugs regularly received no assistance in paying for drugs from insurance or other health coverage. Of this uninsured group, 24 percent incurred out-of-pocket drug expenses in excess of $480 in 1985; the comparable figure for 1986 was 34 percent, a sharp increase from the preceding year (American Association of Retired Persons 1987).

The Pricing of Prescription Drugs

Because many elderly patients pay significant out-of-pocket costs for drugs and because prescription drug prices have increased two to three times faster than all consumer prices since 1981, drug prices have become a source of growing concern for consumers, policymakers, and individual and institutional purchasers. In dollar terms, expenditures for drugs and medical sundries grew from $1.7 billion in 1950, to $3.7 billion in 1960, to $8.0 billion in 1970, to $18.5 billion in 1980, and to $25.8 billion in 1984 (Levit et al. 1985). Costs are expected to rise to $42.4 billion in 1990 (Arnett et al. 1985).

Total drug expenditures depend on the unit price (price per prescription) and the number of prescription drugs dispensed. Prices for drugs at both the producer and retail level rose at rates substantially below the overall inflation rate from the period 1965 to 1974. Between 1974 and 1982, however, prices increased at about the same rate as overall inflation, 7.5 percent.

In recent years trends in drug prices have been changing. Before 1981, prescription drug prices tended to rise more slowly than did the Consumer Price Index—in many years, substantially more slowly. Beginning in 1981, however, prescription drug prices have been rising far faster than the CPI (see Table 5.6). In 1986, for example,

TABLE 5.6

Comparison of Annual Price Changes:
CPI for All Items Versus CPI for Prescription Drugs

Year	CPI for all items	CPI for prescription drugs	Year	CPI for all items	CPI for prescription drugs
1967	—	—	1977	6.5	6.0
1968	4.2%	−1.7%	1978	7.7	7.8
1969	5.4	1.3	1979	11.3	7.8
1970	5.9	1.6	1980	13.5	9.2
1971	4.3	0.1	1981	10.4	11.4
1972	3.3	−0.4	1982	6.1	11.7
1973	6.2	−0.4	1983	3.2	10.9
1974	11.0	2.4	1984	4.3	9.6
1975	9.1	6.2	1985	3.6	9.5
1976	5.8	5.4	1986	1.9	8.6

SOURCE: U.S. Subcommittee on Health and the Environment, Committee on Energy and Commerce, Staff Report on Price Increases for Prescription Drugs and Related Information (July 15, 1985). Data from 1985 and 1986 were obtained directly from the Bureau of Labor Statistics.
NOTE: The price changes from year to year are percentages.

when the overall inflation rate was only 1.9 percent, the drug price inflation rate was 8.6 percent. Thus, for the most recent year for which data were available, drug price increases grew over four times faster than the CPI.

A congressional staff report on price increases in drugs revealed that, between January 1979 and December 1984, those drugs with the greatest price increases were hormones, drugs for diabetics, biologicals (e.g., vaccines), and prescription medica (e.g., syringes, intrauterine devices, diaphragms, etc.), all of which underwent a 102 percent increase. Tranquilizers and sedatives rose 96 percent in price; pain and symptom control drugs, 78 percent; supplements, cough and cold preparations, and drugs for respiratory conditions, 68 percent; circulatories and diuretics, 66 percent; and antiinfective drugs, 58 percent (U.S. House of Representatives, Subcommittee on Health and the Environment 1985).

There may be several reasons why drug companies have significantly increased prices. Revenues are needed, for example, for the introduction of costly new drugs, for their production, and for intensive research and development. Drug companies may also be attempting to compensate for the loss of revenues they have suffered in foreign markets because of the weakening of the American dollar and the increasingly stringent drug price controls in many nations. Price increases in brand-name products may also represent an attempt to compensate for revenues lost because of the growth of the generic market. Some have suggested that the aging of our society is a factor contributing to the rapid increase in drug prices. As noted in the Appendixes, average drug prices for the elderly are higher than those for the rest of the population, probably because the elderly are more likely to take medications for chronic illness, usually given in more doses per prescription than medications for acute conditions. However, analyses presented in the Appendixes suggest that the aging of the population, in and of itself, has not contributed significantly to increased drug prices in recent years.

Other speculation about the reasons for price increases points to the greater incidence of liability—and threat of perhaps much greater incidence in the future—that may compel drug companies to price drugs aggressively to build reserves against potential future losses. There is speculation, too, that the Medicare prospective payment system for inpatient hospital care, implemented in 1983, will depress drug prices in hospitals. This policy may result in lowered profit margins on drugs sold to hospitals, causing drug companies to try to compensate by charging more for drugs sold in retail outlets.

Generic Drugs

A key factor affecting the price of prescription drugs is the current availability of generic drugs from multiple sources, or manufacturers. By selecting a generic-name product that is chemically, biologically, and clinically equivalent to its brand-name counterpart, retail and hospital pharmacists can provide patients with lower-cost drugs. Since the early 1970s, forty-nine states have abolished antisubstitution laws, which restricted the authority of the pharmacist to select from among multisource drugs and dispense an equivalent drug of lower cost to the patient. The laws were changed because of potential cost savings for consumers and because of the belief that pharmacists are more adequately informed than are physicians regarding the therapeutic equivalence of multisource drug products.

Many generic-name drugs are now available from multiple sources, and most are cheaper than their brand-name competitors. Although there are hundreds of producers of generic-name drugs, most such drugs are made by the large pharmaceutical firms that also produce brand-name prescription drugs (*The Economist* 1985). In 1985 generic-name drugs had a market share of 15 to 20 percent, but some analysts predict that market share will increase to 40 percent by the end of the decade (Williams 1985). As a result, the responsibility of the physician in prescribing the lowest-cost clinically equivalent drug and the role of the pharmacist in drug product selection will become increasingly important. The potential for cost savings for the elderly—the largest consumers of drugs—is substantial.

Currently, however, the cost savings that might be achieved by generic-name drug use are not being realized. Physicians are, as a rule, unaware of the availability of equivalent multisource drugs. Consequently, they prescribe higher-priced brand-name drug products in the belief that they are protecting their patients from what they mistakenly believe are lower-quality generic-name drugs. Many physicians do not realize that the Food and Drug Administration reviews information on multisource products before they are marketed and assures their equivalency (Faich et al. 1987). Furthermore, there is a lack of understanding among many physicians of chemical, biological, and therapeutic or clinical equivalence. In 1969 the Task Force on Prescription Drugs defined the terms as follows (U.S. Department of Health, Education, and Welfare 1969):

☐ Chemical equivalents—multisource drug products that contain essentially identical amounts of the identical active ingredients, in identical dosage forms, and that meet existing physiochemical standards in the official drug compendia.

☐ Biological equivalents—chemical equivalents that, when administered in the same amounts, will provide essentially the same biological or physiological availability of the drug, as measured by blood levels, etc.

☐ Therapeutic, or clinical, equivalents—chemical equivalents that, when administered in the same amounts, will provide essentially the same therapeutic effect, as measured by the control of a symptom or disease.

Although these definitions have been adopted by the American Pharmaceutical Association, a significant amount of confusion still exists because of the continued use of the term "generic equivalents." The Task Force did not use that term, but did define both *generic name* and *brand name* as follows (U.S. Department of Health, Education, and Welfare 1969):

☐ Generic name—the established or official name given to a drug or drug product.

☐ Brand name—the registered trademark given to a specific drug product by its manufacturer.

Despite these attempts to clarify the issue, physicians continue to be reluctant to prescribe generic-name drugs. First, brand-name drugs are familiar. Because these drugs are protected from competition by patents which extend for years after the drugs are marketed, brand-name familiarity is established. After a patent expires and a drug becomes available from multiple sources, physicians often continue to prescribe the higher-cost brand-name drug product. The physician is not only already familiar with the brand name, but the generic, or official, name used for the drug may be lengthy and unpronounceable, and, thus, not easily remembered. Second, physicians accept information from drug manufacturers, which is provided through detail persons, advertising, and other promotional vehicles.

Pharmacists, too, are reluctant to exercise authority in drug product selection (Goldberg & DeVito 1983; Goldberg, DeVito & Raskin 1986). Like physicians, pharmacists are influenced by the large drug manufacturers. Furthermore, they do not wish to antagonize local physicians, who might send their patients to another pharmacy if the pharmacist substitutes a generic-name product for a brand-name product. Sometimes, too, they are able to make a greater profit on the sale of a brand-name drug product because the markup on drugs—the amount added by pharmacists to the acquisition cost—is a percentage of the acquisition cost. Thus, the higher the cost of a drug to the pharmacist, the greater the markup or profit per prescription.

In some cases pharmacists try to compensate for lower profit margins on generic-name drugs by charging higher percentage markups for these drugs. They are able to do this because, when the patent on a drug has expired and new manufacturers produce it, the drug is often priced well below the brand-name product. The pharmacist, however, is free to set a higher price if it is to be sold directly to a patient.

Variation in Drug Pricing

The pricing of prescription drugs in the United States is complex and confusing. Pricing involves manufacturers, wholesalers, community pharmacies, both independent and chain stores, hospitals, nursing homes, and federal and state governments. The single most important factor affecting the price of a prescription drug sold in a retail pharmacy is the acquisition cost—the price paid by the pharmacy to the manufacturer, if the purchase is direct, or to the wholesale distributor, if there is an intermediary. Because manufacturers and wholesalers usually give discounts for large purchases, costs will often be lower for hospitals and retail chains than for community pharmacies, which have only modest volumes of prescription drug business.

Price variation for a particular drug may also reflect the different services that pharmacists render to customers. Some pharmacists provide very limited services, simply filling the prescriptions and typing labels on bottles. Other pharmacists provide additional services. They may, for example, monitor nonprescription and prescription drug use by keeping a drug history on the patient; provide information about adverse drug reactions, drug-drug interactions, and drug-food interactions; give advice about drug selection to assure the patient lower cost and equal efficacy when a drug is available from multiple sources; and distribute detailed written instructions to enhance patient compliance.

Like physicians, most community pharmacists would prefer to charge a "usual, customary, and reasonable" price for professional services and for drugs dispensed. Currently the pharmacist's markup— the amount added to the acquisition cost of the drug—is designed to cover the cost of doing business and to provide a profit. In some instances, however, especially when government programs (e.g., Medicaid) are involved, the reimbursement level is fixed and may be below the cost of doing business.

The issue of drug pricing involves not only pharmacies. The prices that are set for drugs sold to hospitals are a source of even greater confusion because of the number of discounts and deals involved. In any case, hospital charges for drugs given to patients, although they may vary from hospital to hospital, are normally a source of substantial revenue above cost. Even more disturbing are charges in nursing homes, where drug overuse appears to be a significant problem and a variety of unsavory practices, including kickbacks by pharmacists to nursing home operators, have been identified (U.S. Senate, Subcommittee on Aging, Subcommittee on Long-Term Care 1976).

Physicians' Knowledge About Drug Prices

Obviously, it is important for physicians to be informed about the prices of the drugs they prescribe. Price is of particular concern to the elderly, for whom out-of-pocket drug expenditures are a significant problem. In addition, Medicare's prospective payment program, involving Diagnosis Related Groups (DRGs), is giving physicians even stronger incentives to reduce drug costs for elderly patients in hospitals. As we have seen, generic-name drugs—drugs that are as effective as, but cost less than, brand-name products—can be prescribed if a physician considers not only appropriate medical care but also cost. Unfortunately, however, physicians are often poorly informed about actual drug prices (Goldberg et al. 1976).

Medical publications that contain information about the benefits of specific drugs do not list prices. These publications include the widely used *Physicians' Desk Reference* and such standard textbooks as Goodman and Gilman's *Pharmacological Basis of Therapeutics*. *The Medical Letter* occasionally provides information on the prices of specific drugs, but it does not do this on a regular basis. Medical journals, such as the *New England Journal of Medicine* and the *Journal of the American Medical Association,* rarely, if ever, include articles that deal with the price of prescription drugs. Nor do physicians routinely consult available resources such as *Facts and Comparisons*, which includes a cost index comparing wholesale prices of similar products within the same therapeutic category, and the *Annual Drug Topics Red Book*, which lists wholesale prices and, often, suggested retail prices for all drugs.

To determine sources that physicians use to inform themselves about drug prices, the FDA sponsored a large-scale survey in 1973. Ten thousand physicians responded, 88 percent of whom listed patient care as their primary activity. Thirty percent of the respondents indicated that they never sought price information at all, whether from peers, advertisements, or articles in journals (Temin 1980). Of the physicians who did try to find out about drug prices, about 25 percent used detail persons as sources of information. The results of this survey, then, indicate that physicians seldom consult informed, disinterested sources and, as a result, rarely have an accurate sense of the costs of the drugs they prescribe.

Protecting the Elderly Against the Rising Costs of Prescription Drugs: Strategies for Action

There are many approaches that can be used to provide the elderly with protection against rising prescription drug costs. Actions can be taken to enhance physicians' knowledge of drug prices and to reimburse pharmacists for their expanded roles in drug product selection and patient counseling. Actions can and are being taken by government at the state and federal levels.

Enhancing Physicians' Knowledge of Drug Prices

If physicians were provided with accurate information about the comparative prices of drugs, the elderly would have some protection against rising costs. Such information could be published in a drug compendium, which was updated at reasonable intervals and gave both clinical and price information for all prescription drugs on the market. The *Guide to Prescription Drug Costs*, published by HCFA in 1980, was designed to serve this purpose (U.S. Department of Health, Education, and Welfare, Health Care Financing Administration 1980). It gave prices for drugs of different brands that have the same therapeutic effect (Lee et al. 1983). The guide was distributed to physicians, hospital pharmacists, and community pharmacists in 1980 but has never been republished.

One disadvantage of a drug compendium is that drug product prices are changing with such rapidity that no such "pricing guide" can ever be completely current. Furthermore, the enactment of the Drug Price Competition and Patent Term Extension Act of 1984 has resulted in numerous brand-name drugs now becoming available in generic form. Prices for these drug products will change rapidly as distributors and manufacturers compete in the marketplace, making it all the more difficult to maintain a current price list that has any degree of accuracy.

It is possible that physicians' knowledge about the comparative prices of drugs may be enhanced in another way. Physicians may simply be forced into educating themselves because of changes in reimbursement policies. As health care plans are shifted from retrospective to prospective payment, there may be far greater incentives for pharmacists participating in these plans to educate physicians about the most cost-effective drugs available, and far greater incentives for physicians to listen to what pharmacists have to say.

Payment to the Pharmacist for Services in Addition to Dispensing

As we mentioned earlier, the pharmacist, by selecting a lower-priced generic-name drug when a higher-priced brand-name drug has been prescribed by a physician, can play a key role in reducing the cost of prescription drugs for the elderly. The opportunity to dispense generic-name drugs will expand dramatically in the next few years because patents have expired on about 160 drugs approved by the FDA since 1962.

If pharmacists are expected to provide a full range of professional services, including selection of drug products, counseling, monitoring of drug use, and record keeping, they should be adequately paid. Instead, pharmacists have faced pressures from government—particularly state governments—to expand their role in drug product selection and patient counseling but to lower their professional fees. In California, for example, the legislature has mandated that pharmacists provide patients with specific information about the possible interaction of any drug with alcohol and also give consultations to patients who request drug information. However, the state made no provision for reimbursing pharmacists for these professional services.

In order to ensure that pharmacists are adequately compensated, we recommend that third-party payers who offer prescription drug benefits reimburse pharmacists for specific professional services in addition to drug dispensing. Elderly patients, particularly, need pharmacists who provide services that go beyond drug dispensing. Many aged people take multiple drugs, and too many of them are taking these drugs in inappropriate, ineffective, and costly ways.

Federal Initiatives to Control Medicaid Drug Expenditures

In 1969 the Task Force on Prescription Drugs first recommended that government payment for prescription drugs should "be based on the cost of the least expensive chemical equivalent of acceptable quality generally available on the market" (U.S. Department of Health, Education, and Welfare 1969: 66). The Task Force estimated that 5 to 8 percent of drugs costs for the elderly could be saved through such a program. These savings seem low because, in 1969, only a few of the prescription drugs in wide use were off patent and available from multiple sources.

In the late 1960s pharmaceutical manufacturers argued vigorously against any attempt by the federal government to limit payment for drugs in the Medicaid program to the lowest-cost chemically equivalent drug on the market. They argued that physicians could not be sure of the clinical equivalence of multisource drug products sold by generic name and that the use of the lowest-cost chemically equivalent drug was tantamount to treatment of the patient based on the price, not the quality, of the drug.

In the 1970s the picture changed rapidly. By 1973, 117 of the 200 most frequently prescribed drugs were off patent, and major pharmaceutical firms had entered the generic-name product market. As more manufacturers entered the market, the prices of generic-name products began to vary widely but were usually well below the price of the equivalent brand-name product (Silverman, Lee & Lydecker 1981). The entry of well-known pharmaceutical manufacturers into the generic-name product market also did much to allay some of the concerns of physicians and pharmacists about the quality of generic-name alternatives. In addition, the FDA developed excellent new manufacturing requirements and bioavailability regulations (Lee et al. 1983). These regulations specified which drugs had bioavailability problems and which did not. The latter drugs could be prescribed or dispensed with the assurance of chemical and biological equivalence.

In 1975 the U.S. Department of Health, Education, and Welfare (DHEW) first issued regulations to establish what has become known as the Maximum Allowable Cost (MAC) program for drugs that are paid for in government-financed programs (primarily Medicaid). The MAC regulations, which became effective in 1976, set the level of reimbursement at the lowest of the following three figures: (1) maximum allowable cost of the drug (as set by the government for selected multisource or generically available drugs), plus a reasonable dispensing fee; (2) estimated acquisition cost of the drug, that is, the price paid by the pharmacist to the wholesaler or manufacturer, plus a reasonable dispensing fee; or (3) the pharmacist's usual and customary charge to the general public for the drug.

Early estimates of potential cost savings by DHEW suggested that there would have been cost savings of $37.2 million in fiscal year 1975 if the MAC program had been in effect and had covered all multisource drugs. These savings were not realized initially, however, because of lawsuits by the Pharmaceutical Manufacturers Association (PMA) and disagreements about implementation of the regulations. So far, the government has assigned official MAC reimbursement levels to only about sixty drugs.

A study by Lee and his colleagues (1983), which made use of both detailed data on fifteen dosage forms on the initial five MAC products in five states and a time series analysis of state drug program data across the states, revealed some potential savings. Projected nationwide savings were between $6 million and $15 million annually.

Despite these favorable projections, actual progress under MAC has been painfully slow. In 1983, HCFA established a task force to review major problems plaguing the MAC program: the controversy surrounding the use of multiple source drugs; the inadequacy of drug reimbursement to pharmacists; and problems in administering the program (e.g., insufficient time allotted to Medicaid agencies to implement MAC limits once they become effective and the inability to raise MAC limits quickly to accommodate changes in the market).

In response to the task force report, HCFA issued a regulation in the *Federal Register* (July 31, 1987) which implemented revised policies that would replace the MAC program. The new policy established two separate upper limits on state Medicaid expenditures for drugs: one limit applies to certain generic drugs (approved by the FDA), and the second limit to all other drugs. These limits are applied on an *aggregate* basis: in other words, HCFA sets aggregate upper limits on the states' total Medicaid payments for drugs rather than placing maximum payment limits on individual drugs, as had been done previously. As a result, state Medicaid agencies will now be able to make higher payments for some drugs and lower payments for others, as long as their total payments do not exceed the upper limits established by HCFA. Under these new regulations, state Medicaid agencies can also experiment with alternative drug reimbursement systems.

Upper limits for certain generic drugs are based on an aggregate payment amount equal to the ingredient cost of the drug, calculated according to a specific formula, and a reasonable dispensing fee. The formula is 150 percent of the least costly therapeutically equivalent drug that can be purchased by pharmacists. (The upper limit established for generic drugs would not apply if the prescribing physician certifies that a brand-name drug is medically necessary.) State payments for all other drugs must not exceed, in the aggregate, the level of payment calculated by applying the lower of (1) the estimated acquisition cost plus a reasonable dispensing fee or (2) the pharmacist's usual and customary charges. The objective of the new policy is to provide flexibility to the states in administering their Medicaid programs. At the same time, the policy is designed to provide savings to the federal government through encouragement of expanded generic drug use. Savings could be obtained for the elderly through a MAC approach to drug costs if out-of-hospital drug coverage were offered as a Medicare benefit and if the number of multisource drugs were to increase.

Expanding Medicare Coverage for Prescription Drugs

What is the federal role in relation to drug costs incurred by the elderly? As we noted at the outset of this chapter, in the years since the enactment of Medicare, many bills were introduced in Congress to expand benefits to include outpatient drugs. None was enacted. However, in the summer of 1987 legislation was proposed in Congress to cover prescription drug spending by Medicare enrollees after the enrollee had met a deductible.

In considering alternative drug insurance proposals, the United States Senate and House of Representatives examined many of the issues identified by Silverman, Lee, and Lydecker (1981) in their analysis of drug insurance options. These issues include selection of beneficiaries; scope of drug coverage (e.g., comprehensive coverage for all drugs versus restricted coverage for so-called maintenance drugs used in the treatment of chronic illness); use of a mandatory or voluntary formulary; use of generic-name products; patient cost-sharing; reimbursement for pharmaceutical services; payment to pharmacists or patients; patient education; and drug utilization review.

The Nature of Drug Coverage

On June 22, 1987 the House of Representatives enacted the "Medicare Catastrophic Protection Act of 1987" (H.R. 2470). Among other provisions for catastrophic coverage, the bill specifies that, effective January 1, 1989, Medicare would cover all outpatient prescription drugs approved as safe and effective by the Food and Drug Administration after the enrollee had incurred $500 in expenses for such drugs in a year.

Medicare would pay participating pharmacies 80 percent of whichever is lower: the actual charges by the pharmacist to the patient or specified limits calculated for each drug. If a generic drug has been approved by the FDA, payment could not exceed the limit for generics, unless the prescribing physician indicated in his or her handwriting that a brand-name drug was medically necessary.

Participating pharmacies would sign an agreement not to charge Medicare patients more than they do the general public, to assist enrollees in determining whether the deductible had been met, and to counsel enrollees on appropriate drug use, drug-drug interactions, and the availability of generic products.

The costs and administration of the drug benefit would be financed by an additional monthly premium paid by all Medicare Part B enrollees (currently about 97 percent of beneficiaries). Additional financing of the drug benefit would come from a supplemental premium, which would be related to the enrollee's income.

On October 27, 1987, the Senate passed its own version of the catastrophic health insurance bill (S. 1127). The House and Senate measures have major differences. The Senate measure would "phase in" Medicare coverage of prescription drugs beginning in 1990. In the first year, Medicare would cover the costs of chemotherapy drugs, immunosuppressive drugs, and intravenous antibiotics. In 1991, coverage would expand to include cardiovascular and diuretic drugs. In 1993, full coverage of drug costs above a deductible would begin with the elderly paying 20 percent of each prescription. The deductible is set at $600 for 1990. Beginning in 1991, the deductible would be increased to reflect increases in the average beneficiary's total spending for drugs. The Senate version places a "cap"—or limit—on what the beneficiary's premium may be in any given year. If the premium in any given year is projected to go beyond these amounts, the Secretary of Health and Human Services is authorized to take steps to reduce overall program costs.

Projected Costs of Extending Prescription Drug Coverage

Some information has been accumulated on the possible cost of extending prescription drug coverage for the elderly not only under Medicare but also under private health insurance (Trapnell 1979). In her analysis of extending outpatient drug coverage for the elderly, Lennox (1979) pointed out the difficulties involved in making accurate estimates regarding the financial impact of the program on beneficiaries, providers, the drug industry, and third-party payers. In particular, it is difficult to predict changes in drug use that might occur because of enactment of expanded Medicare coverage. For persons initially having no coverage for drugs who are then offered full coverage, demand may increase from 50 to 150 percent (Ginsburg & Curtis 1978). (This wide latitude shows the uncertainty involved in trying to project the level of demand induced by additional insurance coverage.) The federal government, in making its estimate of the cost of expanded Medicare coverage for prescription drugs, used an "induction factor" * of 60 percent, which is quite close to the low end of the range presented by Ginsburg and Curtis. Using this factor, the Office of the Actuary, Health Care Financing Administration, estimated that the total cost of the drug insurance program (exclusive of administrative costs) would be $5.8 billion in 1989, $6.3 billion in 1990, $6.8 billion in 1991, and $7.7 billion in 1992.[†] These estimates assume a $500 annual deductible and 20 percent coinsurance for each prescription[‡] on the part of the patient (U.S. Department of Health and Human Services, Health Care Financing Administration, Office of the Actuary 1987b).

We believe that steps to protect the elderly from high prescription drug costs can and should be taken. Extending drug benefits under Medicare is such a step. Recent bills passed by Congress, described above, augur well for the passage of a law giving the elderly some measure of financial security against catastrophic health care costs, including drug costs. As this book went to press, analysts were predicting that the bill would be enacted in 1988.

*The induced cost for prescription drugs represents the additional cost of transferring out-of-pocket payments to a third-party payer (e.g., Medicare). A 60 percent induction factor would work this way: Let's say that before the provision of drug coverage, a person incurred out-of-pocket drug expenditures of $1,500 per year. Assume that an insurance program required an annual deductible of $500. Instead of spending $1,500 out-of-pocket for drugs, the person would now spend the first $500 as out-of-pocket expenditures. After the deductible was met, all subsequent drug costs would be transferred to a third-party payer. In this hypothetical example, the individual had previously spent $1,500; as a result, $1,000 would be transferred to a third-party payer. A 60 percent induction factor means that the transferred cost ($1,000) would increase by 60 percent. Thus, total drug expenditures would be $2,100 ($1,600 plus the $500 deductible).

[†]These estimates can be compared with projected total Medicare outlays. For example, projected total outlays for Medicare for 1989 are $103 billion (U.S. Department of Health and Human Services, Health Care Financing Administration, Office of the Actuary 1987a).

[‡]Coinsurance is the payment of a fixed percentage of the cost of each prescription.

State Programs Providing Assistance for
the Low-Income Elderly

Several states have developed pharmaceutical assistance programs
to protect low-income elderly against out-of-pocket prescription
drug costs. Such programs now exist in New Jersey, Pennsylvania,
Maine, Delaware, Nevada, Rhode Island, Illinois, Connecticut, and
New York. Characteristics of three major programs are described
below.

The New Jersey Program

The first state to implement such a program was New Jersey, in
1978. In that year the state passed legislation setting up a program
that reimburses low-income elderly for outpatient prescription drug
costs. Initially, the program, called the Pharmaceutical Assistance
to the Aged and Disabled Program, was financed solely by general
funds in the state budget. When gambling was legalized, the legislation was changed so that a significant percentage of program costs—
39.5 percent—are now subsidized by casino gambling revenues (New
Jersey Department of Health and Human Services 1987).

The New Jersey program provides that eligible citizens 65 years of
age and older pay $2 toward the cost of each prescription. To prevent
stockpiling of drugs, the plan limits participants to 60 days or 100
doses at one time. Overutilization and underutilization of drugs are
monitored by a computerized drug information system that is maintained by the state's Division of Medical Assistance and Health Services, the agency administering the program. Blue Cross serves as the
fiscal intermediary.

Participating pharmacists are reimbursed by the state for the average wholesale cost of a drug or its regular retail sale price, whichever is
less, plus an average dispensing fee of $3.31 for each prescription
filled. The plan requires pharmacists to fill prescriptions with chemically equivalent generic-name drugs whenever possible. It also requires the elderly participants in the program to pay any difference in
cost between a brand-name drug and its generic-name equivalent if a
brand-name drug product is dispensed.

To qualify for the program, individuals must be New Jersey residents, be at least 65 years of age, and have an annual income of less
than $13,250 for an individual and less than $16,250 for a married
couple. Elderly patients in nursing homes are eligible for the pro-

gram, but Medicaid recipients, because their drug costs are already covered, are not eligible. In 1982 the program was expanded to include the disabled. In 1984, 264,000 people were served by the program at a cost to the state of almost $65 million. In that year the average number of prescriptions per aged recipient was 19.7 (New Jersey Department of Human Services 1985). By fiscal year 1986, there were 239,000 enrollees at a cost to the state of $84 million, and the number of prescriptions per aged recipient was 21. The average cost per aged recipient was $339 (New Jersey Department of Human Services 1987).

The Pennsylvania Program

Pennsylvania's program, the Pharmaceutical Assistance Contract for the Elderly (PACE), was implemented in 1984 under the administrative authority of the Pennsylvania Department of Aging. To be eligible, individuals must be 65 years of age or older and have an income below $12,000 per year for an individual or $15,000 per year for a married couple. Participants in the program pay $4 per prescription. The level of copayment is reviewed regularly by a specially appointed review board, and its amount adjusted to reflect increases or decreases in the cost of drugs. The plan limits participants to purchase of 30 days worth of medicine or 100 doses at one time.

Participating pharmacists are reimbursed by the state for the average wholesale cost of the drug or its regular retail sale price, whichever is less, plus a $2.75 dispensing fee for each prescription filled. Like the New Jersey plan, the Pennsylvania plan requires pharmacists to fill prescriptions with generic-name drugs whenever possible and requires senior citizens to pay any difference in cost between a brand-name drug and its generic-name equivalent if a brand-name drug is dispensed.

Legislators set aside $315 million a year for three years to finance the program. The program is fully funded from profits from the Pennsylvania Lottery and is administered by a private contractor, which handles processing, billing, reimbursement, and maintenance of the data base. By the end of the first year of the program, over 5.5 million prescription drug claims had been filed, at a cost to the PACE program of almost $60 million. The average recipient used 18 prescriptions per year, a number that was projected to grow to at least 22 prescriptions per person per year by 1987 (Pennsylvania Department of Aging 1985). This projection, however, turned out to be an underestimate even by 1986: in fiscal year 1986 there were about 400,000 enrollees in the program using an average of 23 prescriptions per capita. Per capita costs were estimated at $280 per enrollee per year, and total program costs were estimated at $125 million.

The Maine Program

In sharp contrast to the extensive coverage and costs of the New Jersey and Pennsylvania programs, the state of Maine operates a modest program covering a limited number of "life-sustaining" drugs. The plan serves almost 22,000 elderly citizens at an annual cost of $1.2 million. The average cost per client is $55 per year, compared with $160 per client per year in New Jersey (Farley 1982). To save costs, eligibility criteria have been added to an existing tax and rent refund program, thus eliminating the need for separate qualification procedures. In addition, employees of the state Bureau of Taxation administer a portion of the plan during slack periods between income tax collections (Farley 1982).

The primary drawback of the Maine program is that its coverage is restricted to life-sustaining drugs. At present, such drugs are limited to specific drug classes, such as diuretics, digitalis preparations, and antidiabetic agents. The Maine Department of Human Services designates the specific drugs that fall into the "life-sustaining" category. In doing so, it takes into account norms governing good medical practice and the yearly state budget allocation. In 1980 senior citizen groups mounted an effort to have antiarthritics included in the "life-sustaining" category, but the 40 percent increase in appropriations that would have been necessary to finance the change failed to pass the legislature (Farley 1982).

Maine residents eligible for the program are 62 years of age or older and have incomes not exceeding $6,200 for an individual or $7,400 for a household of two or more. Recipients of Medicaid and Supplemental Security Income are excluded. Clients must be certified eligible by the Bureau of Taxation, after which they receive an identification card. Then, the client's only responsibility is a $2 copayment for each prescription received.

Pharmacists receive the copayment from the client and bill the remaining charges directly to the state Department of Human Resources, which provides reimbursement from state funds. Program regulations mandate the use of generic-name drugs when available, and physicians and pharmacists are encouraged to write and fill prescriptions in lots of 100. There is no limit on the number of prescriptions filled for any one person.

Unresolved Issues in State Programs

There has been concern that the number of prescriptions per user, especially in the New Jersey and Pennsylvania programs, is higher than national norms for the noninstitutionalized elderly. As we indicated earlier, the average number of prescriptions for the elderly was estimated to be 17 in 1986 (Waldo 1987). In the New Jersey and Pennsylvania programs, however, the corresponding figures were 21 and 23 prescriptions, respectively. There may be several reasons for the higher use in the state programs. First, there may be a selection bias: people who choose to enroll in a program may be sicker and require more drugs than those who do not participate. Second, the program may enable people who were previously unable to afford necessary drugs to pay for them. Third, because the drug benefit is generous and comprehensive and the amount of the copayment is not excessive, there may be incentives for increased drug prescribing and use.* Fourth, the New Jersey program includes nursing home patients, whose use of drugs per capita greatly exceeds that of the noninstitutionalized elderly.

Whatever the reasons for the high levels of drug use, it is vital from a public health perspective to look beyond them to determine whether the level of use is associated with reductions in morbidity, in use of health care services (especially hospitalization), and in mortality.

*This hypothesis is borne out by the results of a major national randomized controlled trial which examined the effects of different consumer cost-sharing arrangements on the demand for medical care services. The study showed that when consumers paid 95 percent of their drug costs (up to a maximum dollar expenditure), drug expenditures were 57 percent of those incurred by consumers facing no cost-sharing (Leibowitz, Manning & Newhouse 1985).

CHAPTER SIX

Drug Testing, Marketing, and Surveillance: The Role of the Food and Drug Administration

Introduction

Are drugs on the market safe and effective for the elderly? Do the present or the proposed policies of the Food and Drug Administration provide adequate safeguards before drugs are marketed? Is there an effective federal system for monitoring drugs in the elderly after they are marketed to obtain information on adverse effects?

In order to answer these questions, it is important to understand the limits and potential of the FDA's role in the testing, marketing, and surveillance of drugs.

The FDA's Role in the Drug Testing Process: 1938 and 1962 Legislation

Drugs cannot be marketed in the United States without FDA approval. FDA regulations related to drug testing before marketing are based on legislation enacted in 1938 and 1962 and on rulings by the federal courts, including the U.S. Supreme Court (Hutt 1980; Nightingale 1981).

The Food, Drug, and Cosmetic Act of 1938 prohibited the marketing of any new drug for which the manufacturer had not submitted an application to the FDA. A "new drug" (prescription or nonprescription) was defined as (1) any drug not marketed prior to enactment of the 1938 statute, and (2) any drug, regardless of when it was marketed, whose labeling with respect to conditions of use changed or was proposed to be changed, or whose dosage form changed or was proposed to be changed.

Each manufacturer who wished to market a new drug was required to submit to the FDA an application containing reports of investigations made to show that the drug was safe for its intended use. The 1938 Act also specified that drug labeling had to contain adequate directions for use and warnings about possible dangers arising from its use. Before 1962 the sole authority of the FDA, in reviewing a New Drug Application (NDA), related to safety, not effectiveness. Under the 1938 law, the FDA had 60 days after submission in which to review the application. After 60 days, a period which the FDA could extend to a maximum of 180 days, the agency had to reject the application to prevent the drug from being marketed. If the application was not rejected, the drug was considered to be approved.

In 1962 the Food, Drug, and Cosmetic Act was amended. According to the amendments, a manufacturer who wishes to market a new drug is required to submit to the FDA an application containing reports of investigations conducted to show not only that the drug is safe for use but also that there is "substantial evidence" of its effectiveness. (The term "substantial evidence" means evidence derived from well-controlled studies carried out by qualified experts.) Besides augmenting the standards for approving a new drug, the amendments make the FDA into an active participant in the approval process. Instead of allowing a manufacturer's NDA to take effect automatically if the FDA raises no objection, the 1962 amendments require that the FDA give its approval before marketing can begin. The amendments also give the FDA jurisdiction over the testing of all new drugs before they are approved for marketing. A manufacturer has to apply to the agency for approval of its proposed testing procedures.

The New Drug Investigation Process

There are two steps involved in approval of a new drug. The first step involves the Investigational New Drug (IND) process, which pertains to the study of the drug. The second step involves the New Drug Application process, which requires documentation of the drug's safety and effectiveness.

Since 1962, it has been illegal to test in humans an unapproved new drug unless a notice of Claimed Exemption for an IND is filed with the FDA. The IND must contain specific data that supports the safety of the initial use of the drug in human beings, including relevant animal toxicology data and a protocol outlining the planned investigation. The investigation takes place in three phases.

Phase I (Clinical Pharmacology)

This phase is preceded by short-term toxicological studies in animals. The initial studies of the drug's effect in human beings require a small number of people (generally 20 to 80 persons)—many of whom are healthy, but some of whom have the disease or condition for which the drug is intended. It is during this phase that a drug is first used on humans, and the purpose of this part of the clinical investigation is to explore dose ranges, define pharmacologic effects and the doses that cause them, and study the pharmacokinetics (absorption, distribution, metabolism, and excretion) of the drug.

Phase II (First Controlled Studies)

During this phase, experienced investigators conduct controlled clinical trials on a limited number of patients (usually 100 to 200 patients in well-controlled studies) to determine a drug's effectiveness in treatment or prevention of a specific disease. If data from Phase I and Phase II show no problems with safety and indicate effectiveness, large-scale clinical trials commence.

Phase III (Further Clinical Trials)

During this phase, investigators conduct additional controlled and uncontrolled studies of different kinds. Some approximate the medical practice settings—clinics, hospital outpatient facilities, and private practice—in which the drug will be used. Some explore interactions with other drugs, examine dose-response relationships, and develop long-term evidence of safety. Phase III studies, which involve extensive clinical trials encompassing observations of 500 to 3,000 human subjects, are designed to gather additional evidence of a drug's effectiveness for specific indications, to define more precisely its adverse effects, and to identify the best way of using the drug. It should be noted that for less common diseases, Phase III trials are necessarily smaller and, therefore, elicit less information about side effects. The detection of rare adverse effects that occur less frequently than 1 per sample size in the clinical trial (e.g., 1/3,000) is not usually possible in Phase III clinical trials.

The investigations conducted under the IND will provide those data needed to support marketing of the drug or, as may happen, data that show the drug to be ineffective or unsafe. The FDA monitors the studies to be sure that patients are not exposed to undue risk. The sponsor—usually the drug manufacturer—is required to notify the FDA immediately if there are any unexpected severe adverse drug reactions and to take any needed remedial action. An equally important purpose is to ensure that the studies are scientifically well designed and are capable of providing useful evidence about the drug. Further, the FDA often meets with the IND sponsor to consider the kinds of studies that would be needed to gain marketing approval.

Geriatric Drug Testing: Current Status and Proposed FDA Guidelines

The premarket testing of drugs in geriatric populations presents special problems and challenges. Current FDA guidelines point to the need to study a drug "in all age groups, including the geriatric, for which they have significant utility" (Novitch 1983). It had been thought that people over 55 or 60 years of age were generally not included in Phase III clinical trials. However, a 1983 survey by the FDA showed that, in pending and recently approved drug applications, about one-third of the patients were 60 years of age or older and that there was a "reasonable representation of patients in their 70s—generally about 5 to 10 percent" (Novitch 1983). Although older patients were included, it was unusual for a drug sponsor to use the data collected to look for age-related differences in response to the drug in order to determine whether or not special labeling advice was needed when the drug was prescribed for older patients. Also, although patients in their 60s and 70s appeared in trials, still older patients generally did not.

Testing of drugs in the elderly during premarketing drug evaluations can pose scientific and ethical problems. Clinical pharmacologic studies are difficult to perform with elderly subjects because aging is likely to bring about cognitive and sensory changes that may cause variability in measurements of the subjects' responses. In addition, because 80 percent of the elderly suffer from one or more chronic illnesses, most of which are treated with long-term drug therapy, their illnesses and their use of multiple medications may affect the results of tests conducted on new drug products. There is concern, for example, that serious adverse effects might be attributed to the investigational new drug when they are actually related to the patient's disease. Clinical trials attempt to avoid the confounding of study results because of the presence of other diseases, other drugs, and the inclusion of persons who have greater potential for developing new illnesses. Furthermore, IND studies try to establish normal responses to a new drug *before* investigation of abnormal responses. The elderly are more likely to be variable in excretion, metabolism, or in physiological responses—all of which can influence their responses to a drug. (This does not prevent, in any way, an additional study being conducted with elderly who are normal within these parameters.)

Drug testing in the elderly also involves ethical issues that are often not dealt with explicitly. For example, one could argue that when the safety and efficacy of a new drug are unknown, it is not ethical to test the product on a group that is, in general, more debilitated physically—and more likely to have suffered irreversible damage from chronic disease—than are other age groups.

Although the FDA, in 1983, initiated a review of its policies related to premarketing tests of drugs in the elderly, the agency still has not incorporated into its drug testing guidelines the requirement that drugs be tested in this population, even when the drug is likely to be used by a large proportion of the aged. Further, FDA guidelines do not require study of the pharmacokinetics and the pharmacodynamics (dose-effect relationship) of new drugs among elderly patients.

In the early fall of 1983 the FDA made available a "Discussion Paper on Testing of Drugs in the Elderly," a preliminary statement of what the agency eventually intended to propose as formal guidelines (Temple 1983). The draft proposals recommended that the elderly be included in trials of drugs, if they would be exposed to these drugs after the drugs had been approved and marketed. To evaluate these studies, the proposals suggested the use of two screens—a pharmacokinetic screen and an interaction screen.

The pharmacokinetic screen is intended to identify differences in the way drugs are absorbed, metabolized, or excreted. These pharmacokinetic differences have particular relevance for the elderly. The elderly are more likely than are younger people to experience impaired organ function (e.g., kidney, liver, or heart function), to take other medications on a long-term basis, and to undergo changes in lean body weight. Such age-related factors can affect responses to a given dose of a drug. If, for example, an older person takes the same dose of a drug as a younger person, the amount of the drug remaining in the blood could be different, because the elderly person will excrete the drug less rapidly than will the younger person. The response of the older person may differ for other reasons, too. For example, the older person's compensatory mechanisms may be impaired.

A factor that can influence the pharmacokinetics of a drug is the presence of other drugs. The pharmacokinetic screen can be used to evaluate the effects of other drugs on a new drug being investigated.

To administer a pharmacokinetic screen, an investigator obtains one or two blood levels of a drug on all or most patients during clinical trials. A search is then made for associations between unusually high or low blood levels and some other feature of the patient, such as age, existence of kidney failure, or the presence of another drug. For example, one might find that blood levels of a drug, on the average, are three times higher in people with decreased kidney function, but that blood levels are the same, on the average, in both young and old people who have normal kidney function. In that case, dosage must be adjusted for altered kidney function but not for age itself. Alternatively, one might find increased blood levels in all older patients, independent of such factors as kidney, liver, cardiac function, etc. In this case, dosage must be adjusted on the basis of age alone.

The second screen, the interaction screen, is intended to evaluate the effect of a new drug on any other drugs that a patient might be taking. Specifically, the interaction screen can be used to determine whether a new drug affects the blood levels of any other drugs, altering the effectiveness of these drugs. To administer the interaction screen, an investigator measures the blood levels of each drug the patient is taking before he or she uses the new drug. The blood levels are measured again, after the patient has used the new drug for a period of time.

The FDA hoped to complete its guidelines by the end of the summer of 1985, but to date they have not been issued. The completed guidelines will not require that a pharmacokinetic screen be used but will recommend the screen as an optional alternative to specific pharmacokinetic studies in the elderly (Temple 1985). The interaction screen will be retained.

The New Drug Application Process

If manufacturers have completed the investigational phase of testing and have obtained favorable results, they must submit test data to the FDA and seek manufacturing and marketing approval. The New Drug Application must consist of six parts: (1) full documentation of investigations of safety and effectiveness; (2) a full listing of the components of the drug; (3) a full statement of the composition of the drug; (4) a full description of the methods, facilities, and controls used for the manufacturing, processing, and packaging of the drug; (5) samples of the drug; and (6) labeling of the drug. Review of a new drug application can be a lengthy process because the high standards established in the law are reflected in the FDA's regulations and procedures.

Criticisms of the New Drug Application Process

The FDA's critics in industry and the academic community charge that the agency is too slow in reviewing applications, that its requirements for research are not always clear, and that FDA regulations are arbitrary and inconsistent (Lasagna 1984; Wardell 1980, 1981). The FDA, on the other hand, replies that the decisions it must make are extremely complex and have far-reaching impact and that it must act with appropriate caution to protect the public. The agency also places some blame for delays on drug sponsors, pointing out that they are often slow in submitting required materials and that data submitted can be incomplete, poorly presented, or unreliable.

The FDA has responded to some of these criticisms with the New Drug and Antibiotic Regulations, issued in 1985. The regulations are designed to reduce the time required for the FDA to review New Drug Applications by simplifying the application process. Sponsors can now submit tabulations of patient data and an overall report that includes separate technical sections with summaries. These submissions can, in most cases, replace the more lengthy case-report forms. In addition, the new regulations make it clear that the FDA will rely on well-conducted foreign studies (in some cases, as the sole clinical data), improve dispute resolution processes, and alter postmarketing surveillance of new drugs to give higher priority to the detection of serious and unexpected adverse drug effects.

It is premature to speculate about the impact of these regulations on the testing of drugs in the elderly. However, it is the elderly who are most likely to benefit from the postmarketing surveillance regulations, which improve the system designed to detect serious and unexpected adverse effects.

Conditions on the Use of Drugs That Have Met Marketing Requirements

Phase IV Studies

After a drug has been approved and is on the market, the FDA has no direct authority over the way it is used by physicians. The drug may be prescribed for any use that a physician considers appropriate, including uses not approved by the FDA. Once a new drug is in the pharmacy, "The physician may, as part of the practice of medicine, lawfully prescribe a different dosage for his patient, or may otherwise vary the conditions of use from those approved in the package insert, without informing or obtaining the approval of the Food and Drug Administration" (Federal Register 1972; FDA Drug Bulletin 1982).

New uses for drugs appear in medical literature and may become widespread in clinical practice. Some of these uses have proved to be valid while others have not. In some cases these unapproved uses subsequently have been approved by the FDA (for example, propranolol was first approved for cardiac arrhythmias and subsequently approved for angina and hypertension; methotrexate was originally approved for the treatment of cancer and later approved for the treatment of psoriasis).

The FDA has followed a number of approaches designed to control or limit unapproved uses of prescription drugs and to ensure that marketed drugs meet defined standards of quality. The FDA is authorized to require drug manufacturers to establish and maintain records and to report data obtained from clinical experience with drugs. Under this authority, the FDA has required sponsors to supplement their applications, so that certain drugs have to undergo further scientific investigations after NDA approval. The first use of this authority involved the drug levodopa. The FDA rapidly approved levodopa for the treatment of Parkinson's disease, but on condition that the manufacturer conduct long-term studies on safety. Numerous other uses of this authority have followed. For example, in order to obtain approval of cimetidine—a drug used initially for treatment of duodenal ulcers—

the manufacturer agreed to conduct other studies on the drug, such as studies of its safety and effectiveness in the treatment of gastric ulcers, and to carry out a large-scale postmarketing surveillance effort. Generally, industry has agreed to requests for postmarketing surveillance studies and, to our knowledge, there has been no litigation questioning FDA requirements for such studies. Although the FDA lacks authority to require them, these Phase IV studies are almost always performed, because compliance may be a requisite for approval of a drug (U.S. Congress, Office of Technology Assessment 1982).

Labeling Requirements for Drugs

Although the FDA does not directly control physicians' use of drugs, the agency does try to influence prescribing through labeling of prescription drugs. Every new drug marketed is approved with labeling that describes its uses, contraindications, and dosing, gives the warnings and precautions that should be observed, and describes the adverse effects that have been identified. Labeling is made available to physicians and the public through package inserts and information in the *Physicians' Desk Reference*, probably the single book most commonly referred to by physicians. Labeling also represents the basis for advertising; that is, advertising may not contradict the contents of labeling or promote uses of drugs not included in labeling.

In programs related to the labeling of prescription drugs, the FDA has focused attention on the elderly. Under a Labeling Revision Program, the FDA proposed requiring that labeling reflect information about the effects of age on the metabolism, distribution, and excretion of prescription drugs, as well as the relationship of age to adverse drug reactions. To provide prescribers with guidance, the agency's Division of Drug Advertising and Labeling proposed that a section entitled "Geriatric Use" be included in the package insert. The proposed revisions stated that if a specific geriatric indication exists for a drug, it should be described under the "Indications and Usage" section of the package insert and that appropriate dosages for elderly patients should be given under the "Dosage and Administration" section. Finally, if use of a drug by the elderly is associated with a specific hazard, that hazard should be described in the package insert as well (Millstein 1984).

These proposed changes in labeling, as well as the proposed changes in the drug testing guidelines, indicate to the drug industry that it should begin to examine clinical data for patients over the age of 65 years, so that physicians can be warned of potential dangers. For example, if the response to a drug, the incidence of side effects, or the dosage required to obtain optimum response are significantly different in the elderly than they are in younger patients, this information should be stated. Adverse reactions should be examined and documented in clinical trials involving elderly patients. Information about the potential for such reactions should then be placed in the proposed geriatric section of the labeling. If the industry heeds the signals from the FDA and adopts these actions, it would be a significant step forward.

Postmarketing Surveillance: The Role of the FDA in the Reporting of Adverse Reactions

As we have noted, the elderly often take multiple medications simultaneously and often receive drugs for uses that have not been approved by the FDA. Is there any federal system for monitoring drugs after they are marketed to obtain information on adverse effects? The FDA monitors adverse reactions to drugs after they are marketed in many ways, including a spontaneous reporting system (in all cases) and specific epidemiologic studies, where indicated. This is an enormous task, for the agency is responsible for ensuring the safety of 32,000 prescription drugs and 300,000 nonprescription drug products marketed in the United States. Furthermore, over 50 new drugs are approved for marketing each year (Edlavitch, Feinleib & Anello 1985), about 25 of which are new chemical entities (agents not previously marketed in the United States in any dosage form). Because premarketing trials are not likely to detect adverse drug reactions that occur infrequently, the full range of adverse effects must be discovered through postmarketing surveillance.

The FDA's New Drug and Antibiotic Regulations modify the current postmarketing reporting of adverse drug reactions required of drug manufacturers. The primary purpose of this reporting system is to detect potentially serious safety problems with drugs after they are marketed. Under the final rules adopted by the FDA, all adverse drug reactions that are serious and unexpected and any significant increase in frequency of adverse drug experiences that are serious and unexpected will have to be reported to the FDA within fifteen days.

The Division of Drug Experience in the FDA's Bureau of Drugs monitors adverse reactions in several other ways. Through its Spontaneous Reactions Reporting Program, information on adverse drug reactions is sent to the FDA by physicians, pharmacists, and hospitals. The Division also conducts a monthly review of medical literature—reports, letters to the editors of medical journals, etc.—to obtain information on adverse drug reactions. It collects data from contract studies, such as those of the Boston Collaborative Drug Surveillance Program (intensive hospital monitoring) and the Drug Epidemiology Unit at Boston University. It implements in-house monitoring and research studies of data bases, such as those of the Medicaid Medical Information Systems and those of commercial sources of data on drug use. Finally, this department of the FDA collaborates with the World Health Organization by exchanging summaries of adverse drug reactions reported in the previous year (U.S. Congress, Office of Technology Assessment 1982). The FDA currently receives more than 40,000 reports of adverse drug experiences annually from all of these sources.

Each method of monitoring has advantages and disadvantages. For example, spontaneous reporting systems rely on the initiative and willingness of practitioners to observe and report potential adverse effects. Spontaneous reporting systems are effective in detecting acute drug toxicities—those that occur shortly after drug administration—but are less effective in detecting delayed drug toxicities—those that have long-term effects. To discover delayed effects, it is necessary to do formal epidemiologic studies. Formal studies are those in which well-defined populations are studied in terms of drug exposure, clinical outcomes, and a variety of other factors. Such studies are rigorous and systematic but they can be time-consuming and expensive. They may be individual ad hoc studies, including research on a limited number of drugs and diseases, or multipurpose studies, including simultaneous research on drug classes and clinical outcomes. Such studies usually have one of two research designs: (1) a follow-up study directed toward a drug or group of drugs or (2) a case-control study directed toward a specific disease. The FDA uses both of these approaches in contracting work with the Boston Collaborative Drug Surveillance program and the Drug Epidemiology Unit of Boston University.

The present surveillance system has the potential to detect some problems particularly related to the elderly. For example, a 1982 FDA publication, *ADR Highlights*, discussed the association of clonidine (an antihypertensive drug) with hallucinations in elderly patients. Currently, the FDA is analyzing, by age, accumulated reports on adverse drug reactions. In addition, the agency is working with the

American Association of Retired Persons to indicate the drugs that are most likely to cause adverse drug reactions in the elderly and, for each drug, to identify the organ system and the type of reaction involved. As problems are detected, the FDA can make them known to health care practitioners through its channels of communication.

Withdrawal of a Drug from the Market

The federal government has clear authority to remove an approved drug from the marketplace, but, except in unusual cases, the procedure is time-consuming. Ordinarily, the FDA must offer the drug sponsor an opportunity for an administrative hearing. Such a hearing may take many months to conduct and is also subject to judicial review. If, however, a drug constitutes an "imminent hazard to the public health," the Secretary of Health and Human Services may suspend marketing without a hearing. An expedited formal hearing on permanent withdrawal of the drug from the market occurs after withdrawal.

The "imminent hazard" provision has rarely been needed; in cases of obvious risk, sponsors have withdrawn drugs voluntarily. However, it was used in 1977 to remove the drug phenformin from the market (Califano 1981). Most permanent drug withdrawals, however, have been voluntary, albeit sometimes with FDA persuasion. The antiarthritic drug benoxaprofen (Oraflex), for example, was voluntarily withdrawn a few months after its approval in the United States when European experience showed that it could cause fatal liver and kidney failure, especially in the elderly. Similarly, the diuretic Selacryn (ticrynafen), which sometimes caused fatal liver injury, and the antiinflammatory drug Zomax (zomepirac), which caused anaphylactic (severe allergic) reactions, were withdrawn voluntarily—that is, without a formal regulatory procedure.

Prescriptions for Change

Clearly, the FDA has attempted to protect consumers. It could, however, take additional steps to provide even greater assurance of drug safety and efficacy.

The Potential of Multipurpose Automated Data Bases

An important development in postmarketing drug surveillance has been the availability of multipurpose automated data bases, such as those developed in health maintenance organizations. Some exemplary systems are located in the Group Health Cooperative of Puget Sound, a Seattle-based health maintenance organization; the Kaiser Health Plan Permanente Medical Groups in Portland and Los Angeles; the Saskatchewan Prescription Drug Plan in Saskatchewan, Canada; and the Medicaid data base in this country.

Large multipurpose data systems can allow for ongoing systematic collection of an enormous variety of data, including drug exposures, use of inpatient and outpatient health services, patient diagnoses, and clinical outcomes measured over time (an especially important consideration in the elderly, given their burden of chronic illness). Because they have the capacity to provide data on drug use and a variety of patient outcomes, these systems are being used to generate and test hypotheses. The systems are efficient because they are already in place for other purposes and do not require new efforts at data collection. A limitation of these data bases, however, is the difficulty researchers have in obtaining details of individual cases. Furthermore, these systems must be very large to provide data on enough patients so that infrequently occurring adverse drug effects can be detected.

Nevertheless, the FDA should consider the possibility of augmenting its existing systems of postmarketing surveillance by making greater use of multipurpose automated data bases. It is already making extensive use of the Medicaid data base. Collaboration with other systems holds great promise for rigorous, systematic evaluations of long-term drug effects. It is important to note, however, that any proposed augmentation of postmarketing surveillance efforts would require that additional resources be allocated to the FDA for data acquisition, information processing, and establishing linkages among available and emerging drug information systems (U.S. Congress, Office of Technology Assessment 1984).

Premarket Testing of Prescription Drugs
to Be Used Largely by the Elderly

The FDA began, in 1983, to develop guidelines for the premarket testing of prescription drugs that would be used frequently by the elderly. The initial proposal was innovative and "proactive," requiring drug testing in the elderly during Phase II and Phase III testing when the drug under study is likely to be used by a significant number of elderly patients. While industry has already responded to the proposal to a certain extent, the FDA has as yet not taken action on these proposals, and action is long overdue. There is no reason why the FDA cannot adopt guidelines for such testing, just as it has established guidelines for the testing of drugs used frequently by children. There has been a long enough period for review, comment, and revision; we believe that it is time for the FDA to make available a final version of the guidelines and to implement the policies contained in the revised guidelines.

Sources of Drug Information for Health Professionals and Elderly Consumers

PART THREE

Sources of Drug Information for Health Professionals and Elderly Consumers

CHAPTER SEVEN

Education and Sources of Drug Information for Physicians and Pharmacists

Introduction

In 1969 the Task Force on Prescription Drugs, in an attempt to improve drug treatment of the elderly, pointed out that there were inadequacies in the geriatric education of physicians and pharmacists and recommended that curriculum be changed in educational institutions (U.S. Department of Health, Education, and Welfare 1969). Since the report of the Task Force first appeared, major changes have taken place in the education of pharmacists and physicians. However, the attempt to improve geriatric education, especially as it relates to drug prescribing, has not kept pace with the growing needs of the aging population or with developments in pharmacology and pharmacy. There are few programs that adequately prepare physicians and other health professionals for the complex problems that they will encounter in treating the growing number of elderly patients.

In this chapter we describe sources of drug information for health professionals and analyze their adequacy with regard to the elderly. We then identify deficiencies in the current education of physicians and pharmacists and consider some innovative approaches to correcting these deficiencies. Of particular importance are programs that extend the role of clinical pharmacists in providing drug information to practicing physicians.

Drug Information Sources for Health Professionals

The need for information about drugs—adverse reactions, indications, contraindications, interactions, dosage, administration, and warnings—grows more urgent as drugs proliferate in number and type. Although all health professionals should be informed about drugs, the physician, pharmacist, and nurse bear direct responsibility for prescribing, dispensing, and administration. Physicians must know about the special effects of drugs on the elderly: altered dose response and greater likelihood of adverse drug reactions. Nurses' need for information is especially critical if they work in hospitals and nursing homes, whereas pharmacists are responsible for dispensing in these settings as well as in community pharmacies and other retail outlets.

The task of educating physicians, pharmacists, and nurses about prescription drugs is a huge one, for there are over 32,000 prescription drug products marketed in the United States (Edlavitch, Feinleib & Anello 1985). These 32,000 prescription drugs contain over 1,900 active ingredients (Joint Commission on Prescription Drug Use 1980). Since 1940, over 1,000 new chemical entities have been introduced into clinical use, and approximately 50 new drugs are approved for marketing every year. The clinical life span of many drugs is limited by the development of new, more effective, or less hazardous drugs and by the introduction of less costly medicines or new preventive measures; the average market life for a new drug is thought to be about five years. Seventy percent of currently marketed drugs were either unknown or unavailable fifteen years ago. Therefore, those who educate and train health professionals face a formidable challenge. Physicians and pharmacists face a special challenge, for they must keep abreast of developments without being overwhelmed by drug advertisements and promotional material.

Drug Compendia, Medical Journals, and Other Printed Sources

A wide variety of printed sources exist to meet the needs of physicians and pharmacists for drug information. These include FDA-approved package inserts and drug compendia such as the *Physicians' Desk Reference, Facts and Comparisons*, and *AMA Drug Evaluations*. Drug compendia vary in type and scope but generally list a limited number of prescription drugs, giving for each information on chemical and brand name, chemical composition, clinical indications and contraindications, warnings, precautions, interactions, adverse reactions, toxicity, administration, and dosage recommendations. Additional sources include textbooks of basic pharmacology and clinical pharmacology, manuals on medical therapeutics, monographs, medical journals, the FDA *Drug Bulletin* and *The Medical Letter*, and manufacturers' promotional materials.

A physician who pursues information about drug prescribing for the elderly may find a search of the medical literature frustrating; little attention has been paid to this topic. This situation will remain unchanged until greater emphasis is placed on geriatrics in schools of medicine and pharmacy. The problem, however, extends beyond the availability of drug information. In fact, studies indicate that printed sources, when used by themselves, do not have long-term effects on physician prescribing (May, Stewart & Cluff 1974; Schroeder, Caffey & Lorei 1979). Printed matter can reinforce messages communicated through personal visits from sales representatives of pharmaceutical companies (Soumerai & Avorn 1984). As with efforts to improve patient compliance with drug regimen, efforts to improve physician prescribing are most successful when printed materials are accompanied by other more potent interventions, such as face-to-face communication with credible experts (Schaffner et al. 1983; Avorn & Soumerai 1983).

Drug Formularies

A formulary is a published list of pharmaceutical products that have been approved by a body of experts. The purpose of a formulary is to help prescribers and dispensers—usually those working in a hospital setting—to make choices based on rational prescribing, cost containment, or both. Formularies written by physicians convey recommendations for treatment. More often, however, formularies are developed by hospital staff, including physicians and pharmacists, and indicate drug products approved for use in that institution. Health insurance programs, particularly state Medicaid programs, develop formularies to indicate those products for which reimbursement will be allowed. Medicare requires that reimbursement for drugs used in the treatment of hospitalized elderly patients be limited to those included in the *U.S. Pharmacopeia*, the *National Formulary*, and similar standard compendia, or to drugs included in a hospital formulary approved by the hospital's pharmacy and therapeutics committee.

Drug formularies, then, are used in a number of hospitals and can be a valuable source of information for prescribing and dispensing. However, the results of a study at Ohio State University indicate that formularies are used by only about 60 percent of the large nonprofit community hospitals in the United States (Rucker & Visconti 1978). Because it is unlikely that smaller institutions use formularies more frequently than do large hospitals, formularies are probably used by fewer than 50 percent of the community nonprofit hospitals and proprietary hospitals in the United States.

Clearly, there are problems in the use of formularies, even though they meet the need for information about prescription drugs. Many hospitals do not use them. Even when they are used, the large number of drugs or dosage forms included limits their effectiveness. For example, the formularies used by state Medicaid programs include so many drugs that they have been ineffective in controlling the use of less effective preparations. The Ohio State study already mentioned found that those hospital formularies restricting the number of dosage forms for drugs to under 750 were more effective in limiting the use of ineffective preparations than those that had more than 900 dosage forms. Furthermore, the removal of ineffective drugs from a formulary does not deal with the prevalent problem of inappropriate use of effective drugs. Finally, formularies provide general information about drugs, but a physician seeking specific information, particularly about new drugs, must obtain it from other sources.

If these problems could be overcome, the formulary would be a useful means of improving drug prescribing for hospitalized patients. By providing comprehensive drug information to physicians and restricting use in hospitals to those drugs considered the safest and most effective, the formulary can serve as both an educational and a practical tool. The elderly, who use hospitals more frequently than do younger people, obviously would benefit most.

Computerized Drug Information Systems

Although hospitals have installed a number of computerized drug information systems to respond to the immediate need for up-to-date information, the value of such systems is just now being appreciated. Electronic data processing of drug information services has lagged behind other computer applications in hospitals: billing, admissions, accounting, purchasing, inventory control, and medical records have been computerized for years. Despite the lag, many hospitals now have computerized pharmacy systems for inpatient and outpatient services. Dozens of such systems are marketed and used by nonhospital-based drug stores and chain pharmacies, and probably an equal number of systems have been designed for hospital-based pharmacies. The vast majority of hospital-based systems, however, are noncommercial and unmarketed. Some of the systems are quite sophisticated. They can maintain drug profiles, perform inventory control and billing, and identify drug-drug interactions. Some can also monitor drug-disease interactions, drug-laboratory-test interactions (situations in which a drug may affect the result of a laboratory test), and even provide pharmacokinetic calculations to assist physicians in prescribing the appropriate drug. These highly advanced, established systems include the drug information system at Los Angeles County/University of Southern California (USC) Medical Center; the comprehensive hospital-based drug information system in the Latter Day Saints Hospital in Salt Lake City; the drug utilization review program developed for the Group Health Cooperative of Puget Sound, a Seattle-based health maintenance organization; the outpatient drug utilization screening system at the Medical University of South Carolina; and the inpatient drug interaction surveillance system, MEDIPHOR, at Stanford University Medical Center.

The drug information system developed by Maronde and his associates at the Los Angeles County/University of Southern California (USC) Medical Center is designed so that it can be used retrospectively. In other words, it can survey inappropriate prescribing after the fact. It is also used prospectively to forestall problems (Maronde 1977). In the Medical Center's two large outpatient pharmacies, pharmacists can obtain an instant profile of a patient's prescription record, an indication of any known drug allergies, a record of all prescription drugs currently being used, a listing of potential drug-drug interactions, and a disclosure of drug quantities given the patient to determine whether they are of a scale that would suggest a possible suicide attempt or diversion to the street market. Once a pharmacist intercepts a potentially inappropriate prescription, he or she alerts the physician.

The USC computer program matches drug pairs in the patient's drug profile via a drug-drug interaction matrix. When matches are found indicating a possible drug-drug interaction, physicians are alerted and may deal with the problem by modifying the dosage or by selecting a new drug. The system has been extended, for purposes of drug utilization review, to all hospitals and other health care settings under the direct control of the Los Angeles County Department of Health Services.

The system in the Latter Day Saints Hospital in Salt Lake City incorporates many kinds of data and is thus able to provide a relatively broad patient data base. Because it includes the patient's complete medical record, drug monitoring can include not only drug-drug interactions but also drug allergies, drug-laboratory test interactions, and drug-disease interactions. The system can also provide physicians with assistance with specific drug therapies (Hulse et al. 1976). The drug monitoring system developed in 1975 by the Group Health Cooperative of Puget Sound (GHC) is not inexpensive. Over a four-year period, development, maintenance, manpower, and programming time totaled approximately $300,000. Over that same period, however, the system saved about $300,000 a year in salaries, expedited the entire dispensing process, reduced errors, prevented prescribing that might have been irrational or have involved needlessly dangerous drugs, and provided information essential for utilization review (Silverman, Lee & Lydecker 1981). An additional advantage is that it is linked with a system containing data on all GHC hospital discharges and maintained by the Commission on Professional and Hospital Activity Study in Ann Arbor, Michigan. This linkage has made possible the performance of a variety of studies on drug toxicity (Jick 1986).

The drug utilization review procedure at GHC has been rather unusual. It is voluntary and confidential. Every month each physician is privately shown his or her own prescribing pattern along with a statistical analysis of the patterns of peers. Errant physicians may or may not then elect to change their prescribing.

The MEDIPHOR System, an acronym for Monitoring and Evaluation of Drug Interactions by a Pharmacy-Oriented Reporting System, was developed at Stanford University Medical Center in 1973 to monitor drug usage and warn physicians of possible drug interactions in hospitalized patients. An on-line computer-based system informs pharmacists, nurses, and physicians before they administer a dose whether the drug prescribed may cause a clinically significant drug interaction (Tatro et al. 1975). A critical difference between this system and others lies in the data base, which was gathered over a four-year period and is continually updated. It includes only those interactions for which there is documentation in humans that meets explicit criteria of design, quality, and clinical relevance (Blaschke et al. 1981). Moreover, the system offers rapid retrieval of specific drug interaction data and is a useful tool for teaching pharmacists and physicians about drugs. MEDIPHOR is used on-line at Stanford and can also be used to analyze drug profiles from other institutions. These analyses have generated data about prescribing habits and frequency of potential drug-drug interactions in nursing homes. Despite the existence of these sophisticated systems, many computerized systems lack an adequate patient data base. They cannot, then, be broadly applied to give contraindications of specific drugs that may be used in individual patients. Limitations in development and dissemination of computerized drug information systems will, however, probably be overcome during the next decade. Signs of rapid progress are already evident. The American Medical Association has developed a program, GTE-Net, that provides computer access for all types of physicians throughout the country. Information on more than 1,200 generic-name drugs is currently available, and there are plans to add the FDA Drug Alert to the network as well. In addition, five pharmaceutical companies have developed a collaborative project called Phycom, a computer-based drug information system that allows any subscriber to dial for drug information. The continued development and increasing use of such systems should benefit the elderly, who are on drug regimens more complicated than those of other members of the population and are, therefore, at greater risk for adverse drug reactions.

The Role of the Pharmaceutical Industry

The pharmaceutical industry plays a major role in providing information to physicians and pharmacists about prescription drugs. In 1974 researchers at UCSF estimated that 20 percent of the pharmaceutical manufacturer's sales dollar was spent on drug promotion (Silverman & Lee 1974). A 1981 study by the same researchers reaffirmed this estimate, as do other recent studies (Silverman, Lee & Lydecker 1981). Expenditures for promotion range from 15 percent in the United Kingdom to 22 percent in Italy, the Federal Republic of Germany, and the United States (Lee 1981b). In 1981 pharmaceutical manufacturers spent approximately $2.44 billion on drug promotion in the United States (Silverman, Lee & Lydecker 1981). Most of the promotion is directed to physicians; less is directed to pharmacists and dentists, and even less to nurses.

An important part of industry promotion is the *Physicians' Desk Reference (PDR)*, although it is not generally recognized as promotion. Published by Medical Economics, the *PDR* is a compilation of advertising that has been purchased by drug companies to promote brand-name drug products. The *PDR* includes FDA-approved materials that closely resemble approved package inserts. Because there has been little testing of drugs on the elderly, the *PDR*, like package inserts, rarely includes information specifically related to prescribing for the elderly.

Pharmaceutical companies also prepare materials that appear as news reports or articles in newspapers, as scientific articles in professional journals, and as lectures in medical schools. Other promotional efforts, including industry-supported conferences, symposia, and continuing education programs for physicians and pharmacists, provide additional sources of information about drug prescribing.

Most promotion expenditures by the pharmaceutical industry involve advertisements in medical journals, direct-mail advertising, and the use of sales representatives by individual pharmaceutical firms. Visits by sales representatives (detail persons) to physicians' offices appear to have a powerful influence on prescribing. For example, in one study, primary-care physicians who claimed that they were not influenced by sales representatives held beliefs concerning the efficacy of two drug groups (propoxyphene and cerebral "vasodilators") consistent with information received through commercial channels rather than with that received from scientific sources (Avorn, Chen & Hartley 1982).

The role of the industry sales representative, or detail person, has been described as "the foundation for the information process" (Breitman 1986). On the positive side, such representatives are valuable resources for specific information and often assist the practitioner in selecting the right drug product. On the negative side, representatives favor their own products and thus present a biased view. The detail person is often the physician's primary source of information on new drug products (Hemminki 1975). This influence is strong not only in hospitals but also in ambulatory care settings (Temin 1980).

Advertising, too, has a strong effect on physician prescribing. The more a product is advertised, the more it is prescribed. A constant flow of messages that praise brand-name products helps account for the low level of generic prescribing. Advertising also reinforces physicians' inadequate knowledge of indications for and side effects of prescription medications (Lexchin 1986).

The pharmaceutical industry's influence on prescribing is so strong, in part, because medical education, at all levels, fails to explain marketing and promotional practices. Nor do medical schools encourage students to think critically about the industry. When medical students graduate and begin clinical practice as hospital interns and residents, their use of drugs is no longer influenced primarily by medical school lectures and textbooks but by the examples of their senior colleagues, many of whose prescribing preferences were shaped by the drug industry.

The specific methods that are used by the pharmaceutical industry to reach physicians, pharmacists, and others in the provider community have been well documented (Breitman 1986). The process is simple. Physicians are identified by specialty and type of practice (practicing physicians versus those in academic positions) so that companies can target those doctors most likely to prescribe a particular drug product. Once the drug industry obtains this information, it designs messages that are tailored to the type of physician likely to prescribe a given drug. For example, a detail person promoting a particular antibiotic to hospital pharmacists in pharmacy schools or infectious disease specialists in medical schools might urge that a drug be adopted because it is more cost-effective than other agents or because it will not contribute to the development of antibiotic resistance. When discussing the same drug with a cardiovascular surgeon in private practice, however, the detail person might choose to stress that the antibiotic is more effective than are other products in preventing the postoperative infections commonly encountered in this kind of practice.

It is difficult to determine the full extent of the pharmaceutical industry's influence on drug information and education, particularly the continuing education of physicians. However, any strategy to improve physician prescribing that fails to recognize and deal with the influence of the drug industry will have limited effectiveness.

Medical Education

Until recently, the quality of courses in drug therapy for the elderly received scant attention. A survey of 167 educational programs across the country found that, at the medical and graduate student levels, coverage of clinical pharmacology was "moderate," meaning that 50 to 80 percent of the surveyed programs integrated this subject into their training. However, few medical students and residents receive comprehensive training in drug therapy and pharmacology with respect to the elderly (Robbins et al. 1982). This inadequacy in medical schools' training programs reflects the limited time devoted to geriatrics and gerontology (Institute of Medicine 1978). Researchers who recently reviewed the current status of health education with regard to care of the elderly outlined several recommendations (Estes & Weiler 1987):

□ Curricula at all levels should include specialized training in gerontology and geriatrics.

□ Interdisciplinary training should be integrated into gerontological and geriatrics education.

□ Education should be designed to encourage and facilitate empowerment of the elderly.

The relative newness of educational programs in geriatrics and gerontology accounts in large measure for their inadequacy. Other factors are the low priority for these subjects compared with subjects that are more established parts of the curriculum, lack of an adequate knowledge base, absence of adequately trained faculty, ageism or other negative attitudes, and insufficient financing. All in all, it is doubtful that medical schools and programs of graduate medical education will take adequate account of geriatric drug therapy until forced to by the massive demographic shifts occurring in the population.

Pharmacy Education

The education of pharmacists in relation to aged people is also deficient. A 1978 study commissioned by the Bureau of Health Manpower, Health Resources Administration, identified drug-related needs of the elderly and examined geriatrics curricula of eighteen pharmacy schools (U.S. Department of Health, Education, and Welfare 1979). The study generated four recommendations for geriatrics curriculum and resource development:

□ Schools of pharmacy should educate and train their graduates in the basic knowledge, attitudes, and skills needed to meet the pharmaceutical needs of the elderly.

□ Schools of pharmacy should conduct an assessment of their curricula to determine the extent to which course offerings are addressing the needs of the elderly and corresponding functions of pharmacists.

☐ Schools of pharmacy should systematically integrate aspects of aging and care of the aged into existing courses in pharmacy curricula at undergraduate and continuing education levels.

☐ Schools of pharmacy should pursue methods other than traditional teaching or even newly developed methods of clinical training in order to integrate geriatrics and gerontology into the curriculum.

A national survey of all U.S. pharmacy schools was conducted to determine how successfully these recommendations were being implemented. The survey found considerable variation among schools. Twenty-two percent of the nation's pharmacy schools have no geriatric coursework whatsoever, while 35 percent offer courses in which the geriatric content averages less than 12 percent. Forty-three percent of the schools offer courses that focus primarily on geriatrics and often include significant patient contact. The overwhelming majority of schools indicate that they are not developing any geriatric coursework; only four of the sixteen schools that do not offer geriatric coursework now plan to develop it in the near future. Results of this survey reveal that many pharmacy students have no access to adequate training in geriatric pharmacy (Simonson & Pratt 1982).

However, there are new developments that give reason for hope. One such development has been the creation of geriatric curricula and innovative geriatric drug education programs in some schools of pharmacy (Chapter 8). The other involves the formulation of a geriatric curriculum by the American Association of Colleges of Pharmacy (AACP) in 1985 (American Association of Colleges of Pharmacy & Eli Lilly and Company 1985). Several schools have begun integrating the new curriculum into their undergraduate coursework and continuing education programs. For example, the Albany College of Pharmacy offers a course entitled "Pharmacy Practice for the Geriatric Patient." The course is designed for health professionals involved with elderly patients. Upon completion of the lecture series, participants receive a certificate.

The University of Southern California has developed a geriatric "track" to enable its pharmacy students to concentrate on geriatrics while enrolled in the doctoral program. The three-semester program is multidisciplinary and presents information on the demographics of aging as well as pharmacotherapy. The California Pharmacists Association is mounting a statewide effort to educate practicing pharmacists about geriatrics. The Association is offering, based on the AACP curriculum, a continuing education program in geriatrics, leading to a certificate. The program is cosponsored by the state's three schools of pharmacy. The School of Pharmacy at the University of Maryland has established a Center for the Study of Pharmacy and Therapeutics for the Elderly and has pioneered other programs related to geriatric pharmacy education and research.

Physician Education and the Role of Public-Interest Detailers

Pharmaceutical companies have known for years that ongoing, one-to-one contact with physicians by drug company sales representatives delivers a clear and effective message, capable of altering physician prescribing habits (Melmon & Blaschke 1983). Using this knowledge, researchers have made proposals for educating physicians.

Rucker (1976, 1980) first proposed the establishment of a National Drug Education Foundation to provide physicians with objective information from specially trained drug therapy consultants. However, Avorn and Soumerai, in 1983, first reported the results of a study using pharmacists as public-interest detailers, and Schaffner and his colleagues, also in 1983, conducted a similar study using physicians as well as pharmacists. The public-interest detailer, as we have previously discussed, is a highly qualified drug educator who offers physicians up-to-date and unbiased information in an effort to counterbalance the promotional activities of pharmaceutical firms.

In a three-year study Avorn and Soumerai investigated the effects of an educational outreach program in which clinical pharmacists served as academically based public-interest detailers. The study was designed to improve the accuracy and appropriateness of physician prescribing by using person-to-person ongoing communication between physicians and drug therapy consultants. Prescribing from three drug categories involving medications especially susceptible to excessive or inappropriate use was targeted for intervention. Subjects in the study included:

☐ Physicians who prescribed propoxyphene (e.g., Darvon) for routine use as an analgesic instead of prescribing aspirin or acetaminophen.

☐ Physicians who used peripheral and cerebral "vasodilators," frequently prescribed inappropriately for peripheral vascular disease and senile dementia.

☐ Physicians who prescribed the oral cephalosporin cephaloxin (Keflex) in cases in which no antibiotic at all or an older, nonpatented, and less expensive antibiotic would be equally effective.

Over 400 physician prescribers of these drugs were identified through Medicaid records and randomly assigned to one of three groups: a control group, for which there was no intervention; a group that received only printed materials; and a group that received face-to-face education. Results of this experiment revealed that physicians who received unbiased and up-to-date information directly from clinical pharmacists, along with a series of mailed "unadvertisements," reduced their prescribing of the target drugs by 14 percent as compared with physicians in the control group. Between the two groups, a comparable reduction was seen in the number of dollars expended for the drugs targeted in the study. No such behavioral change was seen in physicians who received printed materials only. The effects of the interventions persisted for at least nine months after the inception of the program, with no significant increase in the use of expensive substitute drugs. Thus, academically based public-interest detailing may improve the quality of drug prescribing and reduce unnecessary expenditures.

Researchers in the Schaffner study also found that inappropriate prescribing declined when physicians were visited by physician and pharmacist "detailers" based in medical schools (Schaffner et al. 1983). The investigators conducted a controlled trial of three methods designed to improve antibiotic prescribing in office practice: a mailed brochure, a drug educator (pharmacist) visit, and a physician visit. The drugs in the study were oral cephalosporins and three antibiotics contraindicated for use by physicians in office practice. Medicaid prescribing data were used to target physicians requiring further education about the drugs.

Effectiveness of each method was evaluated by comparing the change in prescribing over the course of a year by physicians receiving education with prescribing by the physicians selected as controls. The mailed brochure had no detectable effect. The pharmacist had only a modest impact, particularly in reducing the average number of contraindicated antibiotic prescriptions written per physician. Physician visits produced the strongest reductions in irrational prescribing. For the contraindicated antibiotics, reductions were 18 percent in number of physicians prescribing; 44 percent in number of patients per physician receiving these drugs; and 54 percent in number of prescriptions written per physician. For the oral cephalosporins, both the number of patients and the number of prescriptions per physician were reduced by 21 percent.

Use of the pharmacist consultant was less effective in the Schaffner study than it was in the Avorn-Soumerai study. In the Schaffner study, physician consultants appeared crucial to generating consistent improvement in prescribing decisions. Several factors may be responsible for the different results of the two studies. Schaffner and his colleagues used only one pharmacist, and the drug educators paid only one visit compared with two visits in Avorn's study. In addition, in Schaffner's study, there was large intergroup variability in prescribing before the intervention, and thus the groups may not have been comparable in the first place. Finally, the training of the drug educators in the two studies differed substantially.

Studies designed to provide such information as the comparative effectiveness of pharmacists and physicians as drug educators are critical because the future of programs developed to educate physicians will rest on the relationship between benefits and costs. Avorn's work indicated that a drug information service based in a medical school would result in net savings; in the Medicaid program, the reduction in unnecessary drug expenditures produced savings greater than the program's costs (Soumerai & Avorn 1986). If the results of these and other studies consistently demonstrate that education programs can be conducted at acceptable cost, there will be strong incentive to create more such programs. Physicians will then have recourse to a clinical, noncommercial public-interest detailer as a reliable source of drug information.

We believe that the large-scale development of public-interest detailing programs provides the best opportunity to improve drug prescribing for the elderly. The advantage of such programs is that they are individualized. In other words, they are tailored to fit the special clinical circumstances facing each physician and his or her reason for prescribing: patient demand, lack of knowledge of alternative therapies, errors of omission, and so forth. The trust that develops through ongoing, direct communication may lead to frank discussion of factors affecting drug use and, hence, to more effective prescribing. Because many physicians are already accustomed to regular visits from representatives of drug companies, they would doubtless welcome consultations with drug educators, whose perspective is broad and impartial.

CHAPTER EIGHT

Innovative Drug Information Programs and Resources for Elderly Consumers

Introduction

The primary sources of drug information for elderly consumers are advertisements for nonprescription drugs in the mass media and information provided personally by health professionals. Messages in the mass media convey information about brand-name nonprescription products and strongly suggest that drugs are an effective means of treating a variety of problems from headaches to hemorrhoids. Many of the messages suggest that if the advertised remedy is not effective, the sufferer should consult a physician. Physicians, pharmacists, and nurses provide individual patients with more specific drug information, which usually concerns a particular prescription drug.

In previous chapters we discussed a number of problems involving the drug information that health professionals provide to elderly patients. We turn our attention in this chapter to consumer-oriented programs and resources that convey needed information to an increasingly receptive elderly population.

The consumer health care movement found an important issue in the area of prescription drug information. In the mid-1970s, a number of consumer organizations filed a petition with the FDA requesting that the agency require patient-directed labeling for prescription drugs (Center for Law and Social Policy 1975). The petition requested the written material be made available to patients at the time that drugs were dispensed by pharmacists. Patient information materials designed to inform consumers about safe and effective drug use became known as patient package inserts (PPIs).

This petition, along with other consumer initiatives, launched major efforts to educate the elderly about drug treatment and use.

Groups across the country developed consumer-oriented drug education programs and resources aimed at providing information directly to elderly patients. Another development involved a major, albeit experimental and short-lived, program that required PPIs for ten drugs that are either commonly used or have narrow risk-safety ratios. Initially developed by the FDA during the Carter Administration, the program was opposed by the American Medical Association, organized groups of retail druggists, and others in the private sector, and was ended early in the Reagan Administration, which favored voluntary efforts at education by drug manufacturers. Consumer demands for comprehensive drug information have also been met by some pharmaceutical manufacturers, who advocate FDA approval of brand-name prescription drug advertising directed to the public. Each of these different approaches to consumer drug education has both advantages and disadvantages for the elderly.

In this chapter we describe the history and current status of these initiatives and analyze their adequacy in meeting the informational needs of our nation's elderly.

Consumer-Oriented Drug Education Programs and Resources

To meet the elderly's need for drug information, community-based programs have been developed in a number of cities across the country. Most of these programs employ group teaching methods. Apart from the primary goal of disseminating information, group teaching also establishes a network to which elderly consumers can turn for help. These community-based programs, which address various consumer groups and use a multitude of teaching methods, may serve as models for the development of other efforts. We shall discuss several of the most innovative programs.

Baltimore: The University of Maryland's Elder-Ed and Elder-Health Programs

At the University of Maryland School of Pharmacy, there are two major drug education programs, based on two distinct educational models. In the first model, Elder-Ed, retired pharmacists are paired with pharmacy students to provide drug education to the elderly at senior centers, senior citizen apartments, and other community sites where elderly citizens congregate. Directed by Dr. Peter Lamy, Professor of Pharmacy at the University of Maryland's School of Pharmacy, the program has been operating since 1979. Start-up funding was provided by the Administration on Aging, and a three-year grant enabled the School of Pharmacy to develop a formal procedure for training second- and third-year pharmacy students and retired community pharmacists. A major objective of the program is the safe and effective use of medicines, the prevention of misuse and abuse of drugs, and the involvement of elderly patients in their own health care (Feinberg 1980a, 1980b).

In addition to providing student-pharmacist presentations at local senior organizations, Elder-Ed has developed innovative instructional materials dealing with topics of special importance to the elderly: nonprescription drugs, generic-name drugs, nutrition and vitamin information, and a personal medication record.

Although Elder-Ed has not been formally evaluated, its effectiveness appears evident in several ways. Community response to the program has been so favorable that similar projects have been developed in other areas of the state. Elder-Ed has also been the basis for programs developed in various cities throughout the Northeast. Program staff have advised pharmacists in Florida, Mississippi, and California on developing similar programs in their states. Thus, Elder-Ed serves as a model for consumer-oriented drug education programs across the country.

One disadvantage of Elder-Ed is that it reaches only those older adults able and willing to attend sessions. Because the program cannot reach a large number of elderly, the University of Maryland School of Pharmacy has developed a second educational model, entitled Elder-Health. Faculty, students, and retired pharmacists train caregivers—professionals and family members—in providing drug services to the elderly in different settings, including the home (Lamy & Feinberg 1982). In this way, the nonambulatory elderly have the chance to obtain valuable information. The Elder-Health program may have a side benefit: younger family members, acting as caregivers, will probably know more than they otherwise would have about the safe and effective use of drugs when they themselves face health problems associated with old age (Lamy & Beardsley 1982).

Elder-Health not only trains care-givers but also establishes long-term relationships between pharmacy students and elderly individuals. Each pharmacy student in the program is required to locate an older person and form a visiting relationship with him or her for three years. During that time, both the student and the senior citizen benefit from the relationship. The student learns about the lives and concerns of older people, and the older person learns about correct use of medications. Students meet with their faculty advisors weekly to discuss their experiences with their elderly associates.

Both Elder-Ed and Elder-Health involve the elderly not only as recipients of drug information but also as providers of such information. By encouraging such exchanges, the developers of these innovative programs hope to bring about change in curriculum, improve the practice of pharmacy, and enhance faculty and student perceptions and knowledge of the drug problems of the aged (Lamy & Beardsley 1982).

San Francisco: SRx—Senior Medication Program

In San Francisco two community health professionals developed, in 1978, a drug education program for the elderly called the Senior Medication Program (SRx). Local foundations provided the funds to launch the program. Initially, the focus was on community pharmacists. Twelve pharmacies were selected to become Health Information Centers for seniors, three in each of four neighborhoods chosen for heavy concentrations of seniors, especially those for whom English was not a first language (e.g., Hispanics, Southeast Asian refugees). Participating pharmacists disseminated drug information in several languages. Each pharmacy in the program also received medical profile cards on which pharmacists recorded elderly customers' medical problems and medications. Thus, if a senior forgot what medication to take or when to take a medication, the pharmacist had a convenient reference source to help the patient (Link & Feiden 1978).

In 1980 the program changed focus: community outreach became the goal. SRx staff visited community sites frequented by seniors. They conducted innovative programs designed to help the elderly improve their use of medications. The program has been integrated into the San Francisco Department of Public Health and now serves as a model for a joint undertaking involving private and public funding sources. The program has four central objectives:

☐ To reduce drug misuse and drug abuse among senior citizens through education on the safe and rational use of medications.

☐ To motivate seniors to become knowledgeable consumers of medications able to take an active role in decisions about their own health care.

☐ To work with and train health care providers to develop strategies for solving problems involving drugs and seniors.

☐ To advocate program, policy, and legislative change.

In addition to providing outreach services to individuals and agencies in San Francisco, SRx has expanded its networking to other counties by establishing a "Regional Outreach Educational Plan." The plan involves six northern California counties which have established organizations similar to SRx and are participating in resource exchange, intercounty use of volunteers, and promotion of policy and legislative change. There is a central regional body that governs the program and supervises the consultation services, the instructional activities, and the educational materials that are used. Each county contributes resources, supplies, and financial and clerical support. Some funding from the California state government also helps support the regional program.

Gardena, California: Medicine Education Program

Another drug education program funded by county government sources is the Medicine Education Program in Gardena, California. Funded by the Los Angeles County Drug Abuse Programs Office, the program delivers services to elderly consumers and their providers within Los Angeles County. The program is part of Behavorial Health Services, a community-based nonprofit agency that has been providing drug and alcohol services since 1973. The Medicine Education Program was started in 1977, soon after the National Institute on Drug Abuse (NIDA) targeted the elderly as a population at high risk for drug-related problems. A series of studies had shown that these drug-related problems result from the misuse and abuse of legally obtainable prescription and nonprescription drugs. In response, NIDA developed a model education program for the elderly, which included booklets and a film describing strategies consumers can use to become rational and informed users of prescription drugs.

Because it provided valuable drug information to the elderly, the NIDA program was considered a useful starting point. However, the founders of the Medicine Education Program believe that information alone, while important, cannot produce behavorial change. Such change, they believe, can be brought about only by an intense educational process that involves the acquisition of skills and values, as well as information, and that provides training in assertive interaction with health providers. The goal is to teach both consumers 50 years of age and older and the service providers who work with them how to prevent medication misuse and how to use the health care system to advantage.

The Medicine Education Program includes a series of four sessions presented throughout Los Angeles County at multipurpose centers, club meetings, retirement residences, church groups, and health centers. The sessions provide information on the effects and correct use of drugs, help seniors to develop techniques for interacting with health care professionals, and suggest actions that can be taken to reduce health risks. There are also extensive written materials, in the form of checklists and fact sheets, that have been designed specifically for use by older adults and have been translated into several languages. These are distributed along with free health materials to each participant for use at home.

Program effectiveness has been evaluated for each year of operation. All evaluations indicate that participants have increased their knowledge of drugs and have undergone positive changes in attitude.

Drug Education Resources

In addition to these community-based drug education programs, there now exist a variety of resources that have been developed to enhance the elderly's knowledge and use of medications. As noted earlier, NIDA developed a film and booklets for older people on the safe use of medications. These educational materials are distributed to state agencies involved in drug abuse prevention. The film, "Wise Use of Drugs—A Program for Older Americans," features physicians, pharmacists, and public health nurses who provide advice and instruction about use of medications. Accompanying the film is a set of booklets that reinforce major points in the movie and serve as resources for older audiences. There is also a Group Leader's Guide to help those who wish to organize workshops.

The American Association of Retired Persons has also developed materials to teach the elderly about the safe and effective use of drugs. This consumer organization distributes a twenty-six-page large-print booklet dealing with problems older consumers confront when taking medicines. Included is a removable "Passport to Good Health" which contains charts on which important drug information can be written. A thirty-minute film is available for use in conjunction with the booklet.

Healthy Older People, a health promotion program for seniors, offers a wide variety of resources to foster safe use of medicines. Sponsored by the U.S. Office of Disease Prevention and Health Promotion and the Administration on Aging, the program has a special coordinator in each state. A Healthy Older People Hotline is available for consumers who want to receive further drug-related information.

This description of consumer-oriented drug education programs and resources is by no means complete; it is meant to give some appreciation of the diversity of efforts in this area. Although the programs and resources differ with respect to organization, staffing, funding sources, sponsorship, and teaching methods, all are innovative efforts to address an important educational need of the elderly.

Patient Package Inserts

A different approach to consumer education, the patient package insert (PPI), is designed to provide the individual patient with information at the time a prescribed drug is dispensed. Patient package inserts are leaflets containing information about a drug's actions, indications, proper use, risks, and side effects. Only in recent years has the idea of providing patients with detailed written information received serious attention in this country.

The Pure Food and Drug Act of 1906, and the amendments made to it in 1912, represented government's first attempts to regulate labeling of drugs. The legislation prohibited manufacturers from making fraudulent and deceptive claims on drug labels. Congress acted further to protect the consumer and to make drug treatment safer when it enacted the Food, Drug, and Cosmetic Act, which we have discussed in Chapter 6. This 1938 legislation established the categories of prescription drugs—those drugs dispensed only with a physician's prescription—and nonprescription drugs—those drugs purchased without a physician's prescription. It also required that both prescription and nonprescription drugs be tested for safety and that nonprescription drugs be given labels containing adequate directions for use, including information about indications, contraindications, and dosage.

Prescription drugs were not required to have the same kind of patient-oriented labeling that was required on nonprescription drugs. Instead, information about prescription drugs was directed to the physician. Since prescription drugs are thought to be safe only if they are prescribed by a physician, instructions for patient use have been considered unnecessary, and even potentially dangerous, because patients might use such instructions to self-medicate inappropriately. As a result, patients have received information about prescription drugs only from physicians and pharmacists or from the simple labels attached to the drug containers.

In recent years, reliance on these methods of communication has been called into question. To ensure that patients receive information essential to safe and effective drug use, the FDA has, for more than a decade, proposed and issued regulations requiring that prescription drugs have labels carrying information that has been especially designed for patients. Regulations requiring consumer-oriented drug labeling have evolved in response to several needs and developments.

When it became clear that the long-term use of certain drugs and devices could have adverse effects, the FDA required that written information be provided to patients receiving isoproterenol inhalators, oral contraceptives, intrauterine contraceptives, estrogens, progestational drug products, and oral postcoital contraceptives. With the exception of the isoproterenol inhalators, all of the consumer-oriented labeling was directed to women of reproductive age and was, in part, the result of widespread public concern about the potential adverse effects of oral contraceptives, intrauterine devices, and estrogens. The provision for patient package inserts was clearly intended to allow patients to participate in the decision to initiate or to continue use of such drugs and devices.

The consumer health movement played a vital role in bringing about the development of PPIs. In 1975 a petition filed with the FDA on behalf of a number of consumer organizations requested that the agency require patient-oriented labeling for all prescription drugs. The petitioners argued that patients have the right to know both the benefits and risks of prescribed medications; thus informed, they are better able to decide whether to initiate or continue use of the prescribed drug therapy (Center for Law and Social Policy 1975). Provision of this information would represent a step toward greater involvement of patients in their own health care decisions and a step closer to informed consent.

Research results corroborate the position taken by the consumer health movement by revealing that patients want information about the drugs prescribed for them (Joubert & Lasagna 1975). Not only do patients want this information but they actually read it. This is particularly true of the aged. A large prospective study of the effects of patient package inserts on patients found that older patients were more likely than were younger people to read the inserts for two of the three drugs studied (Kanouse et al. 1981).

Inappropriate prescribing of drugs has provided another impetus for patient package inserts. These inserts may produce "activated" patients who are able to ask informed questions and thus guide their physicians toward more "rational" prescribing.

The prevalence of noncompliance also shows that there is a need for PPIs. Noncompliance with a drug regimen results, to a large degree, from a breakdown in physician-patient communication. Physicians often do not take sufficient time to explain the drug regimen to patients. Even when a full explanation is given, patients may not understand or may forget oral instructions. As we have already discussed, compliance improves when oral instruction is accompanied by written information.

In 1979 the FDA published in the *Federal Register* a proposal that would eventually have led to the requirement that patient package inserts be developed for most prescription drugs. Organizations representing pharmacists, physicians, and pharmaceutical manufacturers voiced strenuous objections to the proposed program and convinced the FDA to limit its program to a three-year trial period and to ten classes of drugs, many of which are widely used by elderly patients. Final regulations for the pilot program were issued on September 10, 1980. The deadline for manufacturers to develop the first PPIs—for cimetidine, clofibrate, and propoxyphene—was May 25, 1981. PPIs for the other drugs or drug classes—ampicillins, benzodiazepines, methoxsalen, phenytoin, digoxin, thiazides, and warfarin—were to follow. Under this pilot program, patients were to receive PPIs at the time any of the designated drugs were dispensed. Drug manufacturers were required to prepare the leaflets and provide them to pharmacists, who were then required to provide them to patients each time there was a new prescription for one of the drugs. At the end of the three-year period the pilot program was to have been evaluated to provide definitive data about the costs and benefits of PPIs. However, after these final regulations were issued, the Reagan Administration delayed their effective date.

Efforts Involving the Private Sector

Following President Reagan's inauguration in January 1981, the FDA initiated a full review and hearings on patient-oriented labeling of prescription drugs. Based on this review and the Administration's philosophy on regulation, the FDA rescinded the PPI program. One of the reasons given for this decision was the acceleration of voluntary efforts by the private sector to assume responsibility for educating patients. Specifically, the American Medical Association announced its intention to initiate a patient drug education program, the Patient Medication Instruction (PMI) program. The PMI program was designed to develop patient information material for distribution by physicians at the time of prescribing, rather than by pharmacists at the time of dispensing, as proposed by the FDA's pilot program.

Substantial donations from pharmaceutical manufacturers and the AMA's Education and Research Foundation helped launch the program in October 1982. A broad-based marketing campaign was designed to inform physicians about the availability of pads of leaflets providing information on the forty most widely prescribed drugs, many of which are used routinely by the elderly.

Several months following the initiation of the campaign, the AMA tried to determine the extent to which physicians were aware of, understood, and used PMIs. Survey results revealed that 50 percent of the physicians were either unaware of or did not understand what PMIs are. One-third of the physicians who were aware of and understood the purpose of the PMIs actually ordered them, while two-thirds did not. To explain these findings, AMA researchers suggested that physicians who did not use PMIs might be less receptive to new products than were the other physicians (Freshnock 1983). However, it is also possible that physicians failed to order leaflets because they believed that they were already providing adequate drug information to patients, as indicated by FDA-sponsored surveys (Miller 1983).

Overall, 14 percent of the physicians surveyed by the AMA reported regular use of PMIs. When asked specifics about their use, physicians reported that they did not distribute the leaflets to all of their patients but tended to give them to patients they considered to be intelligent and mentally alert. This selective distribution of PMIs is significant. Because the elderly are perceived to be less mentally alert than are younger patients, their physicians may not be giving them this important information. If this is true, it is most unfortunate, because studies show that the elderly need, want, and benefit from written drug information and that the impact of such information is not influenced by alertness, intelligence, or educational level.

In addition to the AMA effort, a group of health professionals, government agencies, pharmaceutical manufacturers, and consumer groups joined with the FDA in forming the National Council on Patient Information and Education (NCPIE). Paul Rogers, former chairman of the House of Representatives Subcommittee on Health and the Environment, chairs the organization. The Council's objective is to improve communication between patients and health care professionals in order to assure safe and effective prescription drug use. It employs public service announcements on television, public and professional education campaigns, a corporate health promotion initiative, a newsletter, and annual meetings. The Council also sponsors special events, like "Talk About Prescriptions Month," held in October 1986. The purpose of these events is to stimulate nationwide and community activity motivating consumers to seek—and health professionals to offer—information on appropriate drug use. These efforts are cosponsored by major consumer organizations, such as the National Council on the Aging.

NCPIE has also been directly involved in addressing drug misuse among the elderly. Using a grant from the Commonwealth Fund, it convened a panel of health and program planning specialists to identify reasons for improper medicine use by older people and to suggest practical approaches for action in priority areas. As an outgrowth of this effort, NCPIE developed a multimedia campaign to improve communication between older consumers and their health care providers. The campaign features public service announcements on television and radio, consumer-patient education brochures, a health care provider brochure, articles written for lay magazines and professional journals, and a planning report entitled "Priorities and Approaches for Improving Prescription Medication Use by Older Americans."

Still another initiative involving the private sector was taken by the United States Pharmacopeial Convention. It has developed two publications, "About Your Medicines" and "Advice for the Patient." These books on prescription drugs are designed for consumers.

Finally, the American Association of Retired Persons (AARP) encloses drug information leaflets with the prescriptions filled through its mail-order pharmacy service. The leaflets, prepared with the assistance and cooperation of the FDA and experts in geriatric medicine and pharmacy, represent a major national voluntary effort by a consumer organization. The program was initiated in May 1982. The nonprofit AARP Pharmacy Service is the world's largest private mail-order pharmacy; it fills more than 7 million prescriptions a year for the elderly. It offers prescription drugs and other health care items to the 28 million members of AARP. Almost 3 million AARP members use the Pharmacy Service each year.

The leaflets prepared by AARP instruct the consumer on how to take particular drugs, provide important facts to remember, describe uses and possible side effects, and explain what the physician needs to know when prescribing. These leaflets have been prepared for the drugs most often used by older persons (e.g., antihypertensive and cardiovascular medications) and are made available to association members at no charge. Seventy-five different leaflets are now available, containing information on more than 300 drugs. A leaflet is provided with each new prescription filled by the AARP Pharmacy Service. Program staff are also exploring ways of disseminating the leaflets to groups that are not part of AARP.

A questionnaire was mailed to 1,650 AARP members who had received leaflets for antihypertensives, tranquilizers, and antiarthritics. Of those who said they received the leaflet, 95 percent read it, 76 percent kept it, and 56 percent discussed it with another person. Respondents taking antihypertensive medicines were apt to have kept the leaflet and said that they obtained new information from it. Those taking tranquilizers most often said that the leaflet raised questions in their minds about their medications and that they discussed the information with their physician (Morris & Olins 1984). These results suggest that the elderly make active use of patient package inserts and that their reactions vary by drug class. When information contained on the drug leaflet creates concerns, the result is increased patient-physician dialogue—precisely the result that medication leaflets are designed to achieve.

Prescription Drug Advertising Directed to Consumers

At the same time that the FDA-supported PPI program was being rescinded and initiatives were being developed by the private sector, some pharmaceutical manufacturers began to advertise brand-name prescription drugs directly to the public via printed advertisements and television commercials. Proponents contended that television commercials and newspaper advertisements inform consumers so that they are able to make intelligent choices. Proponents also argued that advertisements sponsored by drug companies give information on symptoms and available drug treatments and thus help patients to detect and manage their diseases. Opponents argued that such advertisements encourage an unnecessary reliance on brand-name drugs, when, in some instances, exercise, diet, or generic drugs provide safer and less costly alternatives. Opponents also argued that patients lack the expertise necessary to evaluate the claims of prescription drug advertisements and are therefore vulnerable to sophisticated marketing programs. Because these programs have been designed primarily to increase consumption of particular brand-name drugs, they could encourage misuse. Furthermore, opponents pointed out that consumers need objective information about drugs—not the biased information found in printed advertisements and thirty-second commercials. They added that prescription drugs, already very costly, might become even more expensive because the substantial expenses involved in advertising to consumers could be passed on to consumers.

Because of the complexity of this subject and the controversy it provoked, in 1983 FDA Commissioner Hayes called for a moratorium on consumer-oriented drug advertising in which brand names were mentioned. The moratorium was designed to allow the FDA time to study the issue in greater depth. The agency created two "model" prescription drug advertisements which it circulated nationwide. Consumers' reactions were assessed, and survey results helped FDA officials to develop guidelines for drug firms interested in prescription drug advertising aimed directly at consumers.

During the moratorium, many leading drug manufacturers launched major advertising and public relations campaigns designed to encourage consumers to request certain drug products. Although particular brand names were not mentioned in the ads (in compliance with the FDA moratorium), specific diseases for which companies sell drugs were discussed. These advertisements appeared in newspapers and on television stations across the country and have increased the sales of specific drug products (Waldholz 1985).

In 1986 the moratorium was lifted, and more drug manufacturers began testing the waters. For example, Merrell Dow Pharmaceuticals, Inc. went directly to the public with TV commercials and ads in *Time, Newsweek*, and the *Reader's Digest*. The ads asked smokers if they were ready to quit. If so, smokers were told, doctors and Merrell Dow could help. Because the ads did not specifically name Nicorette, the company's prescription gum containing nicotine, Merrell Dow did not need FDA clearance.

The FDA did ask Hoechst-Roussel Pharmaceuticals, Inc. to change TV commercials that were aimed at individuals, many of whom are elderly, suffering from intermittent claudication (inadequate circulation). The FDA objected to the words "medication your doctor can prescribe," arguing that the commercial came close to describing the prescription drug Trental, the only drug approved for this condition. Industry spokespersons view these advertisements as public service announcements, intended to let the public know that treatments are available. However, opposition groups—including the American Association of Retired Persons and the American Medical Association—disagree. They caution that the ads emerging so far may be a step toward product-specific consumer advertising that will not serve the public interest.

Consumer Drug Education for the Elderly: Strategies for Research and Action

Evaluation of Patient Package Inserts

Although the private sector has made laudable attempts to educate consumers about drugs, these attempts should be carefully and critically evaluated. Private sector initiatives have some potential advantages over government-mandated approaches. For instance, they have greater potential for diversity and flexibility and may be more readily accepted by physicians and pharmacists. Such initiatives do, however, have drawbacks. For example, the American Medical Association program of encouraging physicians to distribute leaflets to patients at the time of prescribing is effective only if physicians have the time and the motivation to request the leaflets. The effectiveness of private sector programs should be examined thoroughly. It is essential that we find out what kinds of physicians use patient medication instruction leaflets. Even more important, we must determine whether patients benefit.

Critics of the FDA-sponsored pilot program involving patient package inserts argue that costs would increase if the government were to require that manufacturers provide PPIs. Higher distribution and production costs could lead to higher prices and could also adversely affect incentives for development of new drugs. In addition, if pharmacists were required to provide and explain PPIs, the prices of their services might increase. Thus, federal expenditures for drugs and pharmacist services could grow (U.S. Congress, Office of Technology Assessment 1984).

On the other hand, there are strong arguments in favor of PPIs. First, although studies show that physicians and pharmacists often fail to communicate basic drug information and that patients desire more detailed information, national surveys reveal that the overwhelming proportion of these health professionals feel that they convey adequate drug information to patients (Miller 1983). This belief might prevent physicians and pharmacists from requesting patient medication leaflets that are part of a voluntary effort. Second, if a major purpose of privately sponsored initiatives is to demonstrate that they are at least as effective as federal programs in meeting patients' needs for information, effectiveness can be tested only if both types of programs are implemented, and their results compared. Finally, although opponents of the PPI program object to its potential for escalating costs, they ignore potential cost savings. Such savings could be realized if PPIs—used in combination with oral consultations with a concerned health professional—prevented or reduced drug side effects, interactions, and complications, and decreased drug-related use of health care services, such as hospitalizations and visits to physicians and emergency rooms.

In our view the arguments against FDA efforts to evaluate PPIs are not compelling. The program should have been instituted long ago. It is necessary, however, that any evaluation of PPIs be based on the assumption that drug leaflets, used alone, will not affect compliance. The optimal approach, as we discussed in Chapter 4, is a combination of written information and counseling from well-informed health professionals.

Community-Based Drug Education Programs

We learned of two problems associated with community-based drug education programs as we interviewed program personnel for this book. First, many staff members were unaware of the activities of other programs. Second, for the most part, few rigorous evaluations had been conducted to assess program efficacy. In those instances in which evaluations had taken place, the evaluations were program-specific. As a result, there was no way to compare efficacy across programs.

We suggest that appropriate federal agencies, such as the Administration on Aging and the U.S. Public Health Service, Department of Health and Human Services, join with national organizations on aging, private foundations, and community foundations to conduct a nationwide evaluation of community-based programs providing drug education to the elderly. A first step might involve a meeting of interested officials of all these organizations and the directors of community-based drug education programs. One purpose of the meeting would be the exchange of information. Government officials, leaders in the private sector, and representatives of community-based organizations could share information about drug education efforts at the local level and current initiatives being taken by the private sector. Such a meeting might result in the development and implementation of a mechanism to support effective community-based drug education programs and to evaluate them in a systematic manner. Direct linkages could be established among public agencies, private organizations, and community-based drug education programs. Another purpose of the conference would be the development of large-scale (citywide or regional) drug education programs for the elderly.

Prescription Drug Advertising Directed to Consumers

We have described the efforts being made by pharmaceutical manufacturers to introduce prescription drug advertising directly to the public. Although there is no law or regulation prohibiting such advertising and the FDA has encouraged pharmaceutical companies to make such advertisements candid, balanced, and accurate, we are opposed to direct advertising of prescription drugs to the public.

The problem with such advertising is that it focuses on only one brand-name drug product—the product marketed by the pharmaceutical firm that is paying for the advertising. The benefits and risks of a drug are not analyzed in relation to the benefits and risks of alternative drugs or to therapies that do not involve drugs. Physicians who read drug advertisements have the knowledge to look at the information in a larger context and weigh its merits and drawbacks relative to other available therapies. Most consumers lack this knowledge and cannot, therefore, make informed judgments.

It seems unlikely that the federal government will prohibit direct advertising of prescription drugs to the public, in view of the fact that it lifted the moratorium on such advertising. We suggest, then, the creation of a neutral, nonprofit organization which would have the responsibility of providing balance in the drug-related information reaching the public. If an "equal time" concept were applied, a reasonable portion of the time provided commercial advertising would be set aside for noncommercial patient education messages provided by the new organization (Avorn 1983). Messages could contain thorough analyses of the benefits and risks of alternative drug therapies for a given diagnosis. For example, a comparison could be made of the advantages and disadvantages of the new nonsteroidal antiinflammatory drugs for the treatment of arthritis with the advantages and disadvantages of generic aspirin. Messages could also communicate the information that many problems currently treated with medications could be treated just as well, often more effectively, and certainly far less expensively by methods that do not involve drugs. For example, the most effective treatment for constipation is often a diet high in fiber, adequate fluid intake, and modest exercise. For many patients such a regimen would render chronic laxative use unnecessary. These two examples are especially relevant to the elderly, who are more likely than people in any other age group to be afflicted with arthritis and to be chronic users of laxatives.

Still another antidote to pharmaceutical advertising might be the creation of a publicly funded magazine modeled after *Consumer Reports*. Groups of people with expert knowledge of particular drug classes could be called together to evaluate the relative benefits and costs of drug products. Convenient reference guides could be issued regularly in response to pharmaceutical advertisements appearing in print or on radio and television.

The variety of consumer prescription drug education programs and resources described in this chapter and the intelligence and the concern for effective innovation that they exemplify indicate the commitment of health professionals and the elderly to meet problems with fresh thinking. The situation is encouraging, but programs are still small, local, and experimental. It is necessary to test, refine, and disseminate the best and most effective approaches.

PART FOUR

Drug Policy and Demographics

CHAPTER NINE

Drugs and the Elderly:
Program and Policy Recommendations

Introduction

I n this book we have analyzed the current status of knowledge about drugs and the elderly. We have emphasized the following critical areas of concern.

□ *Research and Education*

Investigators and funding agencies have not paid adequate attention to critical research questions including, but not limited to, the need for drug epidemiology studies in the elderly.

Most medical and pharmacy schools have not developed even minimal programs related to geriatrics in general, and drugs and the elderly in particular.

There is a lack of adequate drug education programs and materials for the elderly.

□ *The Roles and Actions of Health Professionals*

Inappropriate prescribing by physicians leads to inappropriate drug use among the elderly in ambulatory care settings, hospitals, and nursing homes.

The pharmaceutical industry exerts a powerful influence on physician prescribing.

There is poor physician-patient and pharmacist-patient communication with respect to drugs.

The potential of clinical pharmacists to play an active and expanded role in the care of the elderly and in physician education has not been realized.

☐ *Patient Behavior*

Patients' noncompliance with prescribed drug therapy is a major problem having significant clinical and economic consequences.

☐ *Drug Regulation, Economics, and Policy*

Federal guidelines for drug testing in the elderly before the introduction of new drugs into the market are inadequate, and there is a need to augment the current system of postmarketing surveillance.

The prices of prescription drugs have increased rapidly in recent years.

Drug insurance programs do not sufficiently protect the elderly—especially the elderly poor and near-poor—against the financial burden imposed by high drug costs.

In this final chapter, we summarize the issues in geriatric drug use that we consider to be the most urgent. We choose selectively from the significant issues just enumerated. Some areas of concern cannot be resolved directly by changes in programs and policies. There can, however, be significant improvement if our proposals are implemented.

The Need for an Expanded Research Program

Despite the existence of a great deal of information regarding drug therapy and the elderly (especially information gathered in recent years), there is a need for more research. Areas requiring further study include the nature of age-related biological, physiological, and pathological changes; ways in which these changes affect the elderly's response to drugs; and the kinds of drug prescribing, dispensing, and administration appropriate to deal with these changes. An area that has remained virtually unexamined involves the psychological changes (e.g., depression) and social changes (e.g., loss of spouse) that accompany aging and the way they affect the elderly's need for, use of, and response to drugs. Drug epidemiology studies—large-scale studies of drug use and its relationship to clinical outcomes—are urgently needed in elderly populations, especially with regard to psychotropic agents. Private foundations and federal funding agencies (particularly the National Institutes of Health and the Alcohol, Drug Abuse, and Mental Health Administration) should give these areas high priority on their research agendas.

Improving Medical Education

Many health professionals do not like working with elderly patients. Physicians, in particular, have been inculcated early in their training with the belief that "cure" of pathology is the goal of treatment. However, most conditions afflicting the elderly are chronic. By definition, they cannot be "cured." Health professionals must learn that fostering functional independence—enhancing patients' abilities to carry out activities of daily living—is a valuable treatment goal in itself.

Negative attitudes toward the elderly involve more than the inability to cure the aged of chronic disease; they also mirror larger societal stereotypes about aging. Physicians need to be educated about attitudes toward age and about the possible harmful effects of negative attitudes on quality of care. An important aspect of education is information on the specific abilities and potential of the elderly. A foundation can be laid if comprehensive geriatric programs are integrated into medical schools' curricula. Curricular changes should also include emphasis on the principles of geriatric pharmacotherapy and on strategies that physicians can use to prevent, detect, and treat noncompliance by elderly patients.

Strategies to Improve Prescribing by Physicians

Reducing Polypharmacy

Physician prescribing can be compromised by polypharmacy. Strategies for dealing with this problem have been described in Chapter 3. They include, but are not limited to, periodic reviews of each medication in the regimen to determine whether it is still appropriate, whether it is being taken correctly, whether it is having the desired therapeutic response, and whether it is causing any adverse reactions. When an adverse drug reaction is suspected, it may be advisable for physicians to discontinue a patient's drug therapies to determine whether they are causing the adverse reaction. This strategy is highly dependent upon the clinician's judgment that the risks of discontinuing the drugs are justified.

Improving Physician Prescribing in Hospitals
and Outpatient Settings

Changes in physician prescribing for the hospitalized elderly may already be taking place as a result of the prospective payment policies implemented by Medicare in 1983. By providing a fixed payment to hospitals per discharge, the prospective reimbursement system offers incentives to hospitals to reduce not only Medicare patients' length of stay but also the resources used for their care, including drugs. Decreased drug use, of course, does not necessarily lead to improved drug use. Nevertheless, unnecessary use of drugs is both costly and potentially dangerous.

Medical staffs and hospital administrators working under DRGs might consider the conclusions of available research: drug therapy consultants who maintain person-to-person ongoing interaction with physicians provide an effective means of improving physician prescribing. Drug therapy consultants, especially clinical pharmacists, have been effective in monitoring drug utilization and advising physicians about drug choices, especially in hospital settings.

Clinical pharmacists in hospitals can also play a critical role in postdischarge care. Because they have access to physicians, to patients, and to pertinent clinical and diagnostic data, these pharmacists can identify elderly patients at risk for drug misuse (e.g., those patients who, when discharged, are taking several medications). Such patients can then be provided with intensive medication counseling before discharge and at periodic intervals during the critical postdischarge period, when drug-related problems are most likely to emerge. During these consultations, pharmacists can identify drug problems (e.g., dose scheduling and administration difficulties) that may compromise therapy, and then provide appropriate solutions. Pharmacists can also alert patients' physicians to potentially serious drug therapy problems (e.g., drug-drug interactions). This model of care—pharmacists serving as drug therapy consultants for geriatric patients and their physicians—is currently being tested at the El Camino Hospital in Mountain View, California, with funding provided by the John A. Hartford Foundation in New York City.

An alternative proposal—using hospital pharmacists during hospitalization and community pharmacists for follow-up after discharge—also offers promise. Still another proposal would involve the clinical pharmacist as consultant to home health care nurses, who increasingly provide services to the elderly after hospital discharge, and who typically review the drug regimen. Given the complexity of geriatric drug use, this model may improve the quality of care for the elderly in the critical months following hospital discharge, providing a way to monitor patient problems and thus prevent drug-related hospitalizations and emergency room visits.

These approaches are particularly applicable to hospitals that are part of plans with capitated arrangements * for Medicare beneficiaries because such hospitals have incentives to decrease hospital admissions and lower total costs.

Improving Drug Therapy in Nursing Homes

The problem of inappropriate drug use in nursing homes is growing in importance. Nursing home use is projected to increase enormously in coming years: the number of nursing home residents—1.5 million in 1980—is expected to increase to 2.5 million in 2000, an addition of 1,000,000 residents in two decades (Rice & Feldman 1983).

Physicians, pharmacists, and nurses must cooperate to ensure that the elderly in nursing homes receive high-quality care. Such cooperation is imperative if inappropriate drug prescribing, dispensing, and administration are to be avoided. The California experiment, which was described in Chapter 3, provides one model of reform that should be considered for broad-scale testing. In that experiment, pharmacists practicing in licensed health care facilities were permitted to prescribe drugs for patients under protocols established by the facility and with the authorization of the patient's physician.

A significant barrier to pharmacists' assumption of greater responsibility in nursing homes is the absence of any provision for reimbursement. Medicare and Medicaid policies should be changed so that pharmacists can be paid for their prescribing function. However, in order to change federal regulations, it would first be necessary to change state pharmacy practice acts to permit prescribing by pharmacists.

To study the impact of an expanded role for clinical pharmacists in drug prescribing and drug monitoring of elderly patients, researchers

---

* Medicare has a predetermined reimbursement rate to health plans, based upon the age, sex, Medicaid status, and institutional status of enrollees on a county-by-county basis. A health plan, such as an HMO, is capitated when it receives a fixed sum prospectively, regardless of the amount of services that are rendered to the patient.

should implement experimental programs in nursing homes. HCFA could initiate the demonstration projects and then disseminate the results. If the outcomes are positive, HCFA could develop policies and regulations to enable pharmacists not only to prescribe but also to receive reimbursement for prescribing.

It must be emphasized that the "pharmacist-as-prescriber" is only one model among many that could be launched to improve drug prescribing in nursing homes. Other approaches need to be tested as well. For example, geriatric nurse practitioners are playing increasingly important roles in nursing homes. The impact of these practitioners should be assessed.

Drug Regulation, Economics, and Policy

Federal Regulation of Drug Testing in Geriatric Populations

Although the FDA began, in 1983, to explore guidelines for premarket testing of prescription drugs used frequently by the elderly, it has yet to adopt new regulations. The proposed guidelines require drug testing in the elderly during Phase II and Phase III studies (that is, before the drug is released on the market) if the drug under investigation is likely to be used by a significant number of elderly patients. We suggest that the FDA adopt such guidelines, just as it has for drugs used frequently by children. There has been more than enough time for review, comment, and revision. It is time for the FDA to publish the guidelines and to implement the policies contained in them.

In addition, there is need to augment the current broad-based system of postmarketing surveillance—the monitoring of drug safety after a drug is introduced into the market. Several such systems are already in operation. Multipurpose automated data bases, such as those developed by Group Health Cooperative in Puget Sound and Kaiser-Permanente in Portland and Los Angeles, hold great promise for rigorous evaluations of long-term drug effects. Utilization of these or similar data bases could add another useful dimension to the current surveillance system.

Strengthening Pharmaceutical Assistance Programs

Rapidly rising prices for prescription drugs are helping to force the price of drugs beyond the reach of growing numbers of elderly, especially those with limited incomes. To deal with this problem, increasing numbers of states are adopting pharmaceutical assistance programs for the near-poor elderly. These programs give each state flexibility in determining its own funding source, cost-sharing policies, and formulary. In developing the programs, state governments attempt to achieve four goals: access to essential drugs, financial protection for those in greatest need, cost control, and ease of administration. Currently, the costs of state pharmaceutical assistance programs vary widely (Chapter 5). Costs are related to several factors, each of which should be considered by those developing new programs: eligibility criteria (usually determined by income levels); patient cost-sharing provisions (deductibles and/or copayments); use of drug formularies; the nature of the drug product substitution law (whether or not the physician is required to specify in writing that generic substitution is prohibited); and the extent to which physicians and pharmacists favor the use of generic drugs. We suggest that those planning future state initiatives carefully examine each of these factors. We also suggest that the following criteria be considered:

☐ Those qualifying for a state pharmaceutical assistance program should be 65 years of age or older and should be in the poor or near-poor categories (i.e., Medicare beneficiaries living in families whose income is above the poverty level but less than or equal to twice the sum set for the poverty level).

☐ Current programs limit the quantity of any one drug to a 30- to 60-day supply to prevent "stockpiling," or hoarding of drugs. We recommend that this period be extended to 90 days for "maintenance" drugs taken on a regular basis for chronic illness. Our recommendation could control costs by decreasing dispensing fees, reducing claims processing costs, and lowering costs per prescription through volume purchasing. In addition, the system is more convenient for the patient.

☐ States should consider amending existing drug product substitution (DPS) laws to promote prescribing and dispensing of generic drugs. When such laws provide for a two-line prescription form—one line that allows substitution of generic drugs and one that prohibits it— or when the law requires the prescriber to check one of two boxes—

again, one that allows substitution and one that prohibits it—there is a high proportion of prescriptions prohibiting generic-drug substitution. However, when prescribers must indicate in their own handwriting an instruction to the effect that substitution is prohibited (e.g., a statement specifying that the brand-name drug is "medically necessary"), prohibition of generic substitution is exercised very rarely. Without jeopardizing the prescriber's right to prohibit substitution, laws that require prescribers to indicate opposition to substitution in their own handwriting greatly enhance the opportunity for savings through DPS.

☐ Planners of programs should consider instituting formularies, that is, lists of drug entities within which drug substitution is permitted. (Many states have used the formulary adopted by their Medicaid agencies.) Selected nonprescription drugs could be placed on a formulary. For example, if aspirin were listed on a formulary, physicians might be encouraged to prescribe it instead of more expensive—but not necessarily more effective—nonsteroidal antiinflammatory agents. A formularly should contain, too, generic equivalents of drugs used commonly by the elderly (diuretics, digitalis and other cardiovascular agents, antidiabetic drugs, etc.) to encourage cost-effective prescribing. (In states in which generic equivalents of such drugs have not been listed, program costs have been significant—due, in part, to drug expenditures for brand-name products.)

☐ Consideration should be given to developing public-interest detailing programs to enhance drug utilization reviews and quality assurance. Public-interest detailing efforts could be targeted at specific drugs, if inappropriate use is suspected. For example, two H_2 antagonist agents, used for the treatment of peptic ulcers, were among the top ten drugs prescribed in the New Jersey program in 1986 (New Jersey Department of Human Services 1987). Antiulcer drugs are not usually prescribed for elderly patients to such a large extent. Their widespread use in the New Jersey program could indicate that the elderly enrolled in this program are not representative of the elderly population in general, or it could indicate that these drugs are being prescribed for inappropriate indications, including minor gastrointestinal symptoms. Antiulcer drugs could, then, be an appropriate target for public-interest detailing efforts.

Can state pharmaceutical assistance programs improve quality of care while reducing overall health care costs? This question can be answered only if researchers conduct rigorous and systematic studies. However, the cost containment features we have described have the potential to provide savings.

Expanding Medicare Coverage for Outpatient
Prescription Drugs

Rationale for Expanded Drug Coverage

We applaud state pharmaceutical initiatives as short-term local solutions. However, the problem of drug costs for the elderly is not confined to a few states, but is instead a national problem. An elderly
person's ability to pay for outpatient prescription drugs should not depend upon the state in which he or she happens to live. Rapidly escalating prices for prescription drugs are making them inaccessible to
increasing numbers of the elderly. Especially burdened are the poor
who are not eligible for Medicaid* and the near-poor, who incur large
out-of-pocket drug expenses relative to their income.

The elderly's needs for assistance with drug costs can be best met by
a comprehensive federal program that provides out-of-hospital drug
coverage. The recent congressional initiative to expand Medicare by
offering beneficiaries protection against catastrophic health costs, including drug costs, is a promising step. We believe that expanded
drug insurance benefits under Medicare make sense not only in terms
of equity but also in terms of economics. Despite claims that expanding Medicare coverage would dramatically increase federal spending,
there is evidence that drug therapy may actually save money by decreasing morbidity and concomitant use of health care services. Some
studies of specific drugs have shown that these drugs provide eco-
nomical medical therapy and substantially reduce health care costs.
For example, the Pharmaceutical Manufacturers Association (PMA)
sponsored a series of studies to determine the cost-effectiveness of specific drugs. The analyses found that the benefits of pneumococcal vaccine exceeded costs for persons in high-risk groups, such as the elderly
and the chronically ill (Weisbrod & Huston 1983). This conclusion
did not take into account the value of the lives saved by the vaccine.
Researchers also conducted studies of the use of beta-blockers to prevent second heart attacks and to treat glaucoma and angina—all conditions afflicting the elderly (Arthur D. Little, Inc. 1984a, 1984b,
1984c). The use of beta-blockers was compared with the use of nondrug therapies, such as surgery, and with treatment without beta-

* In 44 states the income level for Medicaid eligibility is less than the federal poverty threshold—$5,360 for a single person in 1987 (Hill 1987).

blockers. The researchers reported that the use of beta-blockers produced benefits that greatly exceeded their cost.

Critics of this research may argue, first, that it was sponsored by the PMA—a not-unbiased source. Furthermore, one cannot argue that just because some drugs are cost effective, *all* are. A major national program of expanded drug coverage for Medicare beneficiaries could not be financed *only* by revenues saved through appropriate use of drug therapies.

Objectives for Expanded Drug Coverage

In designing any program for covering out-of-hospital prescription drugs, planners should give consideration to the following objectives:

☐ The primary goal is improved health. Nevertheless, costs of any national drug program must be kept at reasonable levels. The objective is not simply to contain the costs of Medicare or any other individual program. It is to contain the total costs of all health programs.

☐ Patients—especially those with high drug costs and low incomes— must be protected against catastrophic costs of prescription drugs.

☐ Efforts must be made to promote safe and effective drug prescribing. If we simply provide drug benefits to elderly patients—without concomitant incentives to improve geriatric prescribing—we may compound already critical drug misuse problems and add to the nation's mounting health care bill.

☐ The program must be designed so that there is a minimum of rules, regulations, and paperwork.

☐ Pharmacists must receive reimbursement not only for dispensing drugs but also for providing professional consultation services to both geriatric patients and their physicians.

☐ Policies must not discourage the drug industry from supporting productive and innovative research.

☐ Patients must be able to participate in decisions about the drugs they will take and the ways in which they will use those drugs.

Recommendations for Expanded Drug Coverage

Our recommendations, then, for outpatient prescription drug coverage under Medicare can be summarized as follows:

☐ There should be continuation of Medicare's existing prescription drug benefits, including prescription drugs for hospital inpatients and immunosuppressive therapy for one year after organ transplantation. There should be an expansion of Medicare benefits to include coverage for out-of-hospital prescription drugs.

☐ Some form of cost-sharing by patients would minimize overutilization and reduce program costs. Cost-sharing might involve an annual deductible, which would require the patient to pay a fixed amount of prescription drug expenditures per year. Cost-sharing might also include coinsurance—the payment of a fixed percentage of the cost of each prescription.

☐ Program financing could be supported by the inclusion of an additional monthly income-related premium, paid by all Medicare Part B enrollees.

☐ A person who has a yearly income of $5,000 and lacks prescription drug insurance would consider a $400 drug bill catastrophic. People who have low incomes, high drug costs, and no or limited drug coverage are those most in need of protection. To deal with this situation, states might be required, under their Medicaid programs, to pay the additional Medicare Part B premium amounts and to help meet the deductible for the elderly and disabled who have incomes at or below 200 percent of the poverty level. Consideration could also be given to an income-related deductible. Any kind of income-related deductible would have to be examined carefully for administrative and implementation problems.

☐ It is important to put a "cap" (maximum dollar amount) on patients' out-of-pocket health care expenditures (including drug expenditures) to ensure financial protection for those incurring catastrophic costs. This is, after all, the essence of any catastrophic health care coverage.

☐ Federally sponsored studies should be commissioned to obtain information on the costs of expanded drug coverage and the distribution of such costs by beneficiaries' age, gender, income, health status, and health insurance coverage. Policymakers could then use the information to adjust the amounts of deductibles, coinsurance, and premiums. If the costs incurred by the program were either greater or less than projected, the deductible, coinsurance, and premium levels could be altered accordingly. Such information would also enable the Medicare program to direct services to groups most needing them. The drug benefit could then be changed to permit a fairer and more equitable distribution of resources.

☐ Pharmacists providing documented professional consultation services should receive additional and appropriate reimbursement for their services.

☐ Pharmacist reimbursement should be based on the actual acquisition cost of a drug plus a reasonable dispensing fee, appropriately adjusted for inflation.

☐ The processing of claims should involve a minimum of regulations and paperwork. The pharmacist, rather than the patient, should keep records and file claims. The pharmacist should also maintain the patient's records of drug expenditures in order to inform patients when their deductibles have been met. Along with the patient's drug expense records, pharmacists could maintain drug utilization records, which could permit them to monitor serious drug therapy problems, such as drug-drug interactions. Some patients might wish to transfer these drug utilization and expenditure records among competing pharmacies. For this purpose, patients might be given a plastic card having a magnetic tape strip on which expenditure and utilization information has been encoded.

☐ The program should encourage physicians to prescribe appropriately and with due consideration for cost. Incentives should exist for physicians to prescribe and dispense lower-cost, generic-name, chemically equivalent drug products. An incentive that we have already mentioned is the requirement that generic drugs be dispensed unless physicians stipulate in their own writing that a brand-name drug is "medically necessary." In fact, physician prescribing may be affected by another development—physicians' increasing enrollment in capitated health care plans, such as health maintenance organizations. The extension of Medicare to include drug benefits would require HMOs to cover drugs, thus enhancing incentives for physicians to prescribe with cost as well as quality in mind. Such incentives would work especially well when combined with physician-oriented educational activities, such as drug utilization review and public-interest detailing.

☐ Professional review organizations or others should be asked to develop utilization review systems to monitor and evaluate the use of outpatient prescription drugs.

☐ The Medicare program should fund large-scale demonstration projects to evaluate the effectiveness of using clinical pharmacists and physicians as drug consultants to physicians. Public-interest detailing could be performed on a regional basis by medical and/or pharmacy schools under contract with HCFA. If public-interest detailing proves effective on a national scale, it could be integrated into the Medicare program.

If our proposed recommendations are implemented, they have the potential not only to make drugs affordable to a population for whom they are life-saving and life-enhancing technologies but also to improve quality of care and to effect cost savings for elderly patients and for the increasing number of hospitals developing capitation reimbursement systems for the elderly.

Our nation's elders—and our society—deserve no less.

Reference Matter

Drugs and the Elderly: Future Projections

The Authors and Mark S. Freeland

Our policy recommendations have been based on analyses of future developments in our society. Change takes place rapidly. The aging population is growing. New developments in pharmaceuticals occur with frequency. Health care organization and financing are in the process of profound change. Finally, the constant interplay of social, economic, and political factors influences drug use by the elderly.

These factors fall into two broad categories. The first category includes demographic factors, which can be projected with relative accuracy well into the next century. The second involves nondemographic factors, the most important of which concern developments in drugs and changes in health policy and care. Nondemographic factors are far more difficult to forecast. In this Appendix we analyze the probable impact of both sets of factors on geriatric drug use, price, and spending.

Looking into the Future: Demographic Factors

Changes in the Demographic Structure of the Population, 1950–2050

In this section we will examine the impact of population size and its changing age-sex structure on use, price, and spending for prescription drugs while holding all other factors constant (e.g., changes in the economy or organization, financing, and delivery of medical care). Ours is the most comprehensive and detailed analysis to date of the impact of the demographic structure on drug use, price, and spending.

Some of the most significant changes in the population of the United States are associated with the post–World War II baby boom that took place between 1946 and 1964. Baby boomers will begin to reach 65 years of age between 2010 and 2030 and to reach 85 years of age between 2030 and 2050. The increasing number of aged persons and the increasing proportion of aged

TABLE A.I

Historical and Projected Population Figures, 1950–2050

Year	Total population		Population under 65		Population 65 and older	
	In thousands	Pct. change from previous decade	In thousands	Pct. change from previous decade	In thousands	Pct. change from previous decade
1950	157,313	+14.3%	144,712	+12.9%	12,601	+37.0%
1960	188,943	+20.2	171,797	+18.6	17,147	+35.9
1970	214,034	+13.2	193,351	+12.6	20,684	+20.6
1980	235,885	+10.3	209,784	+8.4	26,100	+26.3
1990	258,277	+9.5	225,829	+7.7	32,448	+24.3
2000	277,142	+7.3	240,697	+6.6	36,445	+12.3
2010	293,679	+5.9	252,317	+4.8	41,362	+13.5
2020	307,744	+4.7	253,261	+0.3	54,484	+31.7
2030	317,366	+3.2	249,086	−1.6	68,280	+25.3
2040	323,311	+1.9	252,519	+1.4	70,791	+3.7
2050	326,809	+1.1	255,469	+1.1	71,340	+0.8

SOURCE: Wade 1985.

NOTE: The actuaries from the Social Security Administration make three sets of projections with alternative assumptions for fertility rates, mortality rates, and net immigration. Analyses presented in this Appendix will focus on Alternative II, or Intermediate, projections. Among the three sets of projections, the Intermediate projections are felt to have the greatest likelihood of accuracy. See Appendix B for a description of the assumptions underlying Alternatives I and III and for projections of drug use, price, and spending for these two alternatives.

to nonaged persons are of particular interest to planners and policymakers (Table A.1).

Demographers can more easily project the number of aged persons through 2050 because all such persons have been born by 1985; thus only mortality rates and net immigration—not fertility rates—need to be projected. Our projections are based on Social Security Administration data, which assume a fertility rate of 2.0 (that is, 2.0 births per woman), life expectancy of 76.4 for males and 84.0 for females, and a net annual immigration rate of 500,000 persons (Appendix B, Table B.1).

Population projections corroborate conventional wisdom in some instances while producing surprising results in others.

CONVENTIONAL WISDOM: The elderly population will grow at a higher rate than the nonaged or total populations.

PROJECTION: True. The total population is projected to increase from 235.9 million in 1980 to 326.8 million in 2050, an increase of 39 percent. The population under 65 years of age is projected to grow only 22 percent during this period. The aged population, however, is projected to grow 173 percent, from 26.1 million in 1980 to 71.3 million in 2050. In other words, persons aged 65 or over constituted 11 percent of the population in 1980 but will make up 22 percent in 2050.

CONVENTIONAL WISDOM: The rate of growth of the elderly population will be higher in the future than in the past.

PROJECTION: False. Surprisingly, the aged population grew at a faster rate during the period from 1940 to 1980 than is expected for the period from 1980 to 2050. Even during the peak projected growth period of 2010 to 2020, when the increase in the number of elderly is expected to be 32 percent, the growth is lower than the 37 percent for the period 1940 to 1950 and the 36 percent for the period 1950 to 1960 (Table A.1).

However, in *absolute* terms the growth in the elderly population will be substantially higher. Because of the size of the aging baby boom population, the 13.1 million increase in aged persons during the decade 2010 to 2020 is nearly four times greater than the 3.4 million increase in elderly during the decade 1940 to 1950 (Appendix B, Table B.6).

CONVENTIONAL WISDOM: The ratio of aged persons to nonaged adults will continue to grow.

PROJECTION: True. The rapid increase in the percentage of population that is aged will result in an increase in the aged or gerontic dependency ratio—the ratio of aged persons to persons 20 to 64 years of age (Appendix B, Table B.5). The gerontic dependency ratio rises sharply between 2010 and 2030, reflecting the fact that the baby boom population reaches 65 years and older during this period. The gerontic dependency ratio doubles between 1980 and 2030, rising from 19.4 percent to 39.6 percent (Appendix B, Table B.5). Between 2030 and 2050, this ratio is relatively flat.

The gerontic dependency ratio has great significance for Medicare, Social

TABLE A.2

Number of Prescriptions Per Capita, Average Charges Per Prescription, and Average Charges Per Capita, by Age Category, 1977

Age category	No. of prescriptions per capita			Ave. charges per prescription			Ave. charges per capita		
	Females	Males	Total	Females	Males	Total	Females	Males	Total
Under 65	4.4	2.7	3.6	$5.76	$5.96	$5.84	$25.58	$16.69	$21.12
65 and over	12.1	8.6	10.7	$6.47	$7.05	$6.66	$77.16	$57.43	$69.25
Total	5.4	3.2	4.3	$5.96	$6.21	$6.05	$32.03	$20.25	$26.25

SOURCE: Unpublished tabulations from NCHSR National Health Care Expenditures Study.

NOTE: The data were tabulated with five-year age intervals and smoothed using the Whittaker-Henderson type B graduation procedure (Miller 1946); see Table B.7.

Security, and other programs for the aged that are financed primarily by the working population. A larger proportion of aged in relation to working persons places an increasing tax burden on the working population to finance benefit payments for the retired.* Attempts to ensure the economic and social well-being of both of the groups—the working and the retired—will probably result in evolutionary changes in economic, political, and social policy (e.g., increasing the age at which Medicare eligibility begins).

Projections of Drug Use, Price, and Spending, 1950–2050

A summary of drug use and drug charges by sex for the aged, nonaged, and total populations is presented in Table A.2.† On average, aged persons use 10.7 prescriptions per capita per year, whereas the nonaged use 3.6 prescriptions per capita. Females tend to obtain more prescriptions per capita than do males; aged females (12.1 prescriptions per capita) obtain 40 percent more prescriptions per capita than do aged males (8.6 prescriptions per capita). The 1977 average charge per prescription of $6.66 for elderly persons is 14 percent higher than the $5.84 charge for the nonaged. In 1977 elderly persons had an average charge per capita of $69, more than triple the $21 for the nonaged. Charges per capita of $77 for aged females are 34 percent higher than charges of $57 for aged males.

As the size and age-sex structure of the population change, the changes affect not only programs such as Social Security and Medicare but also drug use, price, and spending. To analyze that impact, we have, using 1977 as a base year, projected drug use forward to 2050 and backward to 1950. In calculating the projections, rates of use and charges by age and sex were held constant at the 1977 level. Thus, our estimates are not projections of what will actually happen, but rather projections of what would happen to drug use and charges *if* all that changed were the size and age-sex composition of the population. This approach permits the effects of age to be evaluated independently of changes in nondemographic factors, which we will examine later.

---

* The rising gerontic dependency ratios, especially beginning early in the next century, raise serious questions about the employment of the aged, Social Security financing, and private pension policies. These issues are beyond the scope of this book. For analyses of the economic and social implications of the increasing gerontic dependency ratios, see Siegel and Taeuber (1986).

† The data base used for estimating prescriptions per capita, charges per prescription, and charges per capita by sex and age is the National Center for Health Services Research National Health Care Expenditures Survey. The rationale for the choice of this 1977 household survey and the detailed unpublished tabulations of use, charges per prescription, and charges per capita by sex for five-year age intervals is presented in Appendix B.

TABLE A.3

Historical and Projected Number of Prescriptions, Total Index and Per Capita, for the Total Population, 1950–2050

	No. of prescriptions			
Year	Total index (1977 = 100)	Pct. change from previous decade	Per capita	Pct. change from previous decade
1950	66.0	+19.6%	4.2	+4.3%
1960	80.1	+21.4	4.2	+1.2
1970	91.6	+14.4	4.2	+1.0
1980	104.7	+16.0	4.4	+3.3
1990	118.4	+13.1	4.5	+3.7
2000	133.1	+12.4	4.8	+4.6
2010	148.6	+11.6	5.0	+5.5
2020	163.3	+9.9	5.3	+4.8
2030	173.9	+6.5	5.4	+3.2
2040	178.4	+2.6	5.5	+0.7
2050	179.3	+0.6	5.4	−0.5

Table A.3 gives the data on projected prescription drug use, based on the size and age-sex composition of the total population in the period 1950 to 2050. Table A.4 gives the same data for the elderly. Not surprisingly, growth in the aggregate number of prescriptions for the total and aged populations is quite closely associated with the growth in these populations. (Compare population growth rates in Table A.1 with growth rates in aggregate number of prescriptions in Tables A.3 and A.4.)

Surprisingly, the most rapid increases in aggregate number of prescriptions for both total and aged populations have already taken place. However, it is important to remember that growth in the absolute number of aged persons will be much higher in future decades (Appendix B, Table B.6). Thus, there will be a substantial increase in the number of prescription drugs used in the future, even though the *percentage* growth will be lower.

For most of the decades between 1950 and 2050, growth in the size of the total population has a substantially greater impact on use of drugs than do changes in the age-sex composition of the population. However, for the period between 2000 and 2030, age-sex factors will account for nearly half of the growth in number of prescriptions for the total population (Table A.3). For the aged population, changes in the age-sex composition have little effect; the growth in number of prescriptions is accounted for by changes in the size of that population (Table A.4). Based solely on the size and demographic composition of the population, prescription drug use is expected to

TABLE A.4

Historical and Projected Number of Prescriptions, Total Index and Per Capita, for the Population 65 and Over, 1950–2050

		No. of prescriptions		
Year	Total index (1977 = 100)	Pct. change from previous decade	Per capita	Pct. change from previous decade
1950	50.5	+37.9%	10.4	+0.6%
1960	69.3	+37.2	10.5	+0.9
1970	84.8	+22.4	10.7	+1.4
1980	107.3	+26.5	10.7	+0.2
1990	133.4	+24.3	10.7	+0.0
2000	150.2	+12.6	10.7	+0.3
2010	168.6	+12.3	10.6	−1.1
2020	220.2	+30.6	10.5	−0.8
2030	277.8	+26.2	10.6	+0.7
2040	289.2	+4.1	10.6	+0.4
2050	288.1	−0.4	10.5	−1.1

grow almost three times faster for the aged than for the nonaged (Table A.4 and Appendix B, Table B.8).

Tables A.5 and A.6 present total, per capita, and per prescription charges for prescription drugs for the period 1950–2050 for the total and elderly populations. As with the number of prescriptions, growth in total charges (in constant 1977 dollars) for prescription drugs is quite closely associated with growth in the total and the aged populations. (Compare population growth rates in Table A.1 with growth rates in aggregate constant dollar charges in Tables A.5 and A.6).

Changes in the age-sex structure of the population have a very small impact on average *charge* per prescription for the total population in the period from 1950 to 2050. For the aged population, there is essentially no impact. Consequently, almost all of the changes in per capita spending reflect the impact of changes in age-sex composition on per capita *use*.

The Relative Importance of Demographic and Nondemographic Factors

Although demographic factors are of considerable interest to planners, nondemographic factors—including those that are subject to control by policymakers, such as coverage of outpatient prescription drugs, and those that are not, such as prescription size—may be of greater importance. In this

TABLE A.5

Historical and Projected Total and Per Prescription Index Charges, and Per Capita Dollar Charges, for Prescription Drugs for the Total Population, 1950–2050

Year	Total index (1977 = 100)	Pct. change from previous decade	Charges for prescription drugs (constant 1977 dollars)		Per prescription index (1977 = 100)	Pct. change from previous decade
			Per capita dollar amount	Pct. change from previous decade		
1950	65.6	+19.7%	$25.02	+4.7%	99.1	+0.4%
1960	79.6	+21.3	25.27	+1.0	99.2	+0.1
1970	91.4	+14.8	25.61	+1.3	99.6	+0.4
1980	104.4	+14.2	26.55	+3.9	100.1	+0.5
1990	119.0	+14.0	27.63	+4.1	100.5	+0.4
2000	134.8	+13.3	29.17	+5.6	101.3	+0.8
2010	151.5	+12.4	30.94	+6.1	102.1	+0.8
2020	167.2	+10.4	32.59	+5.3	102.9	+0.8
2030	178.4	+6.7	33.71	+3.4	103.4	+0.5
2040	182.8	+2.5	33.92	+0.6	103.4	+0.0
2050	183.6	+0.4	33.69	−0.7	103.3	−0.1

TABLE A.6

Historical and Projected Total and Per Prescription Index Charges, and Per Capita Dollar Charges, for Prescription Drugs for the Population 65 and Over, 1950–2050

Year	Total index (1977 = 100)	Pct. change from previous decade	Charges for prescription drugs (constant 1977 dollars)		Per prescription index (1977 = 100)	Pct. change from previous decade
			Per capita dollar amount	Pct. change from previous decade		
1950	50.7	+37.8%	$67.85	+0.5%	100.6	−0.1
1960	69.5	+37.1	68.35	+0.7	100.4	−0.2
1970	84.9	+22.2	69.15	+1.2	100.1	−0.3
1980	107.2	+26.3	69.25	+0.1	100.0	−0.1
1990	133.3	+24.3	69.21	−0.1	100.0	0.0
2000	149.7	+12.3	69.23	0.0	100.0	0.0
2010	168.0	+12.2	68.46	−1.1	100.1	+0.1
2020	219.9	+30.9	68.02	−0.6	100.2	+0.1
2030	277.4	+26.1	68.46	+0.6	100.3	+0.1
2040	287.8	+3.7	68.51	+0.1	100.1	−0.2
2050	286.2	−0.6	67.18	−1.9	100.1	0.0

TABLE A.7

Total Number of Prescriptions, Population, and Age-Sex Index of Prescription Drug Use Per Capita, Selected Years, 1970–85

	1970	1975	1980	1985
Total prescriptions[a]	1,279,872,000	1,489,856,000	1,394,337,000	1,548,412,000
Total population	214,034,498	224,483,655	235,884,745	247,423,760
No. of prescriptions per capita[b]	6.0	6.6	5.9	6.3
Age-sex index of prescription drug use per capita (1977 = 100)[c]	97.9	99.3	101.1	102.8
No. of prescriptions per capita deflated by the age-sex index of prescriptions per capita[d]	6.1	6.7	5.9	6.1

SOURCES: IMS America, Ltd.; Wade 1985.

[a]Total prescriptions are usually reported in the April issue of Pharmacy Times.
[b]Total prescriptions divided by total population. Note that the Social Security Area Population includes some persons not included in the IMS America, Ltd. data base. This results in a slightly lower per capita number of prescriptions, but the trend in number of prescriptions should not be significantly affected.
[c]Division of National Cost Estimates, Office of the Actuary, Health Care Financing Administration, Baltimore, Md., unpublished. Also see Table A.3.
[d]This series reflects the number of prescriptions per capita after effects of age and sex have been factored out.

section, data on total number of prescriptions and average charge per prescription are used to illustrate the relative contributions of demographic and nondemographic factors to the growth in total number of prescriptions, prescriptions per capita, and average charge per prescription from 1970 to 1985 (Tables A.7 and A.8). The data pertain to the entire population, because separate data on the aged and nonaged are not available. Total number of prescriptions grew from 1.3 billion in 1970 to 1.5 billion in 1985 (Table A.7) for an average annual growth rate of 1.3 percent. This rate is only slightly higher than the 1 percent average annual growth in total population for this same period.

The average annual growth rate in per capita number of prescriptions was approximately 2 percent for the period 1970 to 1975, whereas the average annual rate declined by 2 percent for the period 1975 to 1980. For the most recent period, 1980 to 1985, the average annual rate in per capita number of prescriptions increased by about 1 percent.

The age-sex index of prescription drug use per capita increased steadily but at a much lower annual rate of approximately one-third of 1 percent during each of the subperiods. The average annual rate of change in number of prescriptions per capita *not* accounted for by shifts in the demographic composition of the population varies substantially from period to period (Appendix B, Table B.14). For the most recent period, 1980 to 1985, the average annual rate of increase in prescriptions per capita not accounted for by changes in age-sex composition was slightly less than 1 percent.

The relative contributions of demographic and nondemographic factors to the growth in total prescriptions vary substantially from period to period (Appendix B, Table B.14). During the period from 1970 to 1975, growth in total population accounted for 31 percent of growth in total number of prescriptions (Table A.9). Changes in age-sex composition accounted for 9 percent of the growth in total prescriptions, and changes in nondemographic factors accounted for 60 percent of the growth. For the most recent period, 1980 to 1985, total population accounted for 46 percent of growth in total prescriptions, age-sex composition accounted for 16 percent, and nondemographic factors (e.g., changes in physicians' prescribing patterns, changing prescription size, changes in health coverage for prescription drugs) accounted for 38 percent. When the effects of total population and age-sex composition are combined, demographic factors account for 62 percent of the growth in total number of prescriptions during this period.

Although demographic factors have had a significant impact on total number of prescriptions, nondemographic factors can also greatly affect awareness by consumers, physicians, and pharmacists that certain prescription drugs may have harmful side effects either in themselves or in combination with other drugs or alcohol. Such awareness can lead to decreased use of such drugs.

In contrast to drug use, drug charges per prescription have not been sig-

TABLE A.8

*Average Charge Per Prescription, Consumer Price Index for Prescription Drugs,
and Age-Sex Index of Average Charge Per Prescription, Selected Years, 1970–85*

	1970	1975	1980	1985
Average charge per prescription[a]	$4.02	$5.20	$7.66	$13.10
CPI for Prescription Drugs (1967 = 100)	101.2	109.3	154.8	256.5
Deflated average charge per prescription[b]	$3.97	$4.76	$4.95	$5.11
Age-sex index of average charge per prescription[c] (1977 = 100)	99.6	99.9	100.1	100.3
Residual deflated charge per prescription[d]	$3.99	$4.77	$4.94	$5.10

SOURCES: IMS America, Ltd.; Bureau of Labor Statistics.

[a]Average charges are usually reported in the April issue of *Pharmacy Times*.

[b]Average charge per prescription deflated by the Consumer Price Index for Prescription Drugs.

[c]Division of National Cost Estimates, Office of the Actuary, Health Care Financing Administration, Baltimore, Md., unpublished. See also Table A.5 and Table B.7 in Appendix B.

[d]Deflated average charge per prescription divided by the age-sex index of average charge per prescription. This category reflects the impact of factors other than changes in the age-sex mix and prescription drug price inflation (CPI for Prescription Drugs) on growth in average charge per prescription—for example, changes in the prescription size and the mix of drugs not associated with demographics.

nificantly affected by demographic factors. Average charge per prescription has more than tripled between 1970 and 1985, rising from $4.02 to $13.10 (Table A.8). This results in an average annual rate of increase of 8.2 percent (Appendix B, Table B.15). This increase reflects a combination of factors, including, most importantly, the increase in the Consumer Price Index (CPI) for Prescription Drugs, which holds constant the average prescription size and the mix of therapeutic categories (i.e., the types of drugs used). In addition, average charges per prescription are also influenced by changes in prescription size as well as changes in therapeutic mix (Appendix B, Table B.15). The CPI for Prescription Drugs increased at an average annual rate of 6.4 percent during the period from 1970 to 1980. Average charge per prescription, controlling for the increase in the CPI for Prescription Drugs, increased at an average annual rate of 1.7 percent.

For the period 1970 to 1985, the increase in the price per dose for a fixed market basket of prescription drugs (as measured by the CPI) accounted for 79 percent of the increase in the average charge per prescription (Table A.10). This underscores the major role of prescription drug price inflation

TABLE A.9

Factors Accounting for Growth in Total Number of Prescriptions, Selected Years, 1970–85

Factors	Relative proportion of factors accounting for growth				
	1970–75	1975–80	1980–85	1970–80	1970–85
Total	100.0%	[a]	100.0%	100.0%	100.0%
Total population	31.3	[a]	45.6	113.5	76.2
Age-sex index of prescriptions per capita[b]	9.2	[a]	16.1	37.3	25.7
Other per capita[c]	59.5	[a]	38.3	−50.8	−1.9

SOURCES: IMS America, Ltd.; Wade 1985.

NOTE: For derivation of method used to allocate factors, see Arnett, McKusick, Sonnefeld & Cowell 1986.

[a] Due to negative growth in total prescriptions during this period, the relative contributions cannot be calculated.

[b] Division of National Cost Estimates, Office of the Actuary, Health Care Financing Administration, Baltimore, Md., unpublished. See also Table A.3 and Table B.7 in Appendix B.

[c] "Other" is a residual and can be interpreted as changes in prescriptions per capita not accounted for by the age-sex index of prescriptions per capita. This factor includes the influence of changes in insurance, income, prescribing practices, regulations, and so forth. Because each of the individual factors is measured imperfectly, "Other" should be interpreted cautiously.

TABLE A.10

Factors Accounting for Growth in Average Charge Per Prescription, Selected Years, 1970–85

Factors	Relative proportion of factors accounting for growth				
	1970–75	1975–80	1980–85	1970–80	1970–85
Total	100.0%	100.0%	100.0%	100.0%	100.0%
Prices[a]	29.6	90.1	93.1	66.0	79.0
Age-sex distribution[b]	1.1	0.6	0.4	0.8	0.6
Other[c]	69.3	9.3	6.5	33.2	20.4

SOURCES: IMS America, Ltd.; Wade 1985.

NOTE: For derivation of method used to allocate factors, see Arnett, McKusick, Sonnefeld & Cowell 1986.

[a] Consumer Price Index for Prescription Drugs.

[b] Division of National Cost Estimates, Office of the Actuary, Health Care Financing Administration, Baltimore, Md., unpublished. Also see Table A.5.

[c] "Other" is a residual and can be interpreted as changes in real spending per prescription not accounted for by the age-sex index of average charge per prescription. This factor includes changes in the mix of prescription drugs and changes in prescription size. Because each of the individual factors is measured imperfectly, "Other" should be interpreted cautiously.

(CPI for Prescription Drugs) in the rising average charge for prescription drugs. Since 1975, the Consumer Price Index for Prescription Drugs has accounted for 90 percent or more of the rise in the average charge per prescription (Table A.10).

Changes in the demographic composition of the population have had a minuscule effect—1 percent or less—on the increase in average charge per prescription for the period 1970 to 1985. This finding undermines the prevailing belief that the aging of the population has had a substantial impact on increasing charges per prescription.* (This belief derives from the view that growth in the aging population results in greater use of more expensive drugs and therefore in higher average charge per prescription for the entire population.)

After we have eliminated the effects of drug price inflation (the CPI for Prescription Drugs) and changes in the age-sex composition of the population, the residual factors accounted for 69 percent of the growth in average charge per prescription for the period 1970 to 1975, but only 9 percent and 7 percent, respectively, for the periods 1975 to 1980 and 1980 to 1985. The basic findings are clear: price inflation for the period from 1975 to 1985 was the dominant determinant of the increasing average charge per prescription rather than changes in prescription size and mix of drug categories. Furthermore, the changing demographic composition of the population has little impact on the average charge per prescription. The impact of other factors—especially changes in prescription size and changes in the mix of drug categories—was more important for the period 1970 to 1975 than for the period 1975 to 1985.

Looking into the Future:
Nondemographic Factors

In addition to drug price inflation, a number of other nondemographic factors will influence drug use per capita and average charge per prescription. The most important of these factors are developments affecting drugs directly and changes taking place in health policies and care.

Developments Affecting Drugs and Their Use

One development affecting drugs is a trend toward the conversion of prescription drugs to nonprescription status. Experts have predicted that the

---

* Because this result is different from what was anticipated, we developed an age-sex composition index for average charge per prescription using the 1980 Health Care Financing Administration and National Center for Health Statistics, National Medical Care Expenditure and Utilization Survey. It produced essentially identical results.

FDA will accelerate such conversion (Bezold et al. 1984). Those in favor of conversion believe that many prescription drugs contain relatively innocuous ingredients. Examples of such drugs are Benadryl and Motrin, which can now be marketed as nonprescription drugs. Proponents of conversion also point out that there is an increasingly educated and medically sophisticated public, capable of self-administration of drugs. Not surprisingly, the pharmaceutical industry wants brand-name products moved to nonprescription status when patent protection expires. The drugs can then be advertised directly to the public, and sales expanded.

If a number of prescription drugs are converted to nonprescription status, the unit price of some drugs may decrease because of increased competition among manufacturers. Another effect will be the enhanced importance of the pharmacist, who is frequently asked for advice about nonprescription drugs.

Another development concerning drugs—the proliferation of generic products—has already been discussed in Chapter 5. Some analysts predict that by 1990 the market share for generic drugs will reach 40 percent, up from 15 to 20 percent in 1985 (Williams 1985). However, availability of generic drugs does not ensure their use. Fears about the safety and efficacy of these drugs are widespread among physicians, pharmacists, and consumers. There is a need for educational efforts, preferably initiated by the FDA, to counteract the drug industry's campaign against generics—a campaign that intensified following passage of the Drug Restoration and Patent Term Extension Act of 1984. In any case, changes in the financing and distribution of health services and drugs will probably accelerate the prescribing of generic drugs, their dispensing by pharmacists, and their use by consumers. Should this occur, the result will be reductions in average charge per prescription and total drug spending per capita. Savings for the elderly could be significant.

A third development likely to occur is the introduction of increasingly effective but expensive drugs. Because many of these drugs will be designed especially for patients with heart disease, this development will particularly affect the aged (Bezold et al. 1984). New prescription drugs for other chronic diseases, such as diabetes mellitus and osteoarthritis, are also forthcoming. The new drugs will probably be priced higher than the prescription drugs now used to treat these diseases. The reason for higher prices is that a company that develops a new drug has, for a time, a monopoly in the marketplace. In addition, the company must price the drug high enough to recover research and development costs (Comanor 1986).

A more significant effect of the introduction of new drugs, however, could be higher quality, better economy, and improved outcomes in health care for the elderly. Because drugs are probably the most cost-effective method of managing chronic disease, effective drug therapy can produce substantial savings in the costs of health care by decreasing morbidity and eliminating the need for more expensive forms of medical treatment, such as hospitalization.* Use of drug therapy can not only reduce health care expenditures, but it can also prevent suffering, disability, and needless death. Safe and effective prescribing and use of antihypertensive regimen, for example, can prevent strokes and heart attacks, with all of their attendant "costs": lost productivity, lost wages, direct medical care costs, and diminished quality of life. Of course, the use of drugs to treat diseases for which no effective therapy previously existed can increase health care costs, provided the drug costs are higher than the costs of prior therapeutic methods.

The fourth development concerning drugs regards drug price increases relative to the growth in the income of the elderly. Drug prices are projected to outpace increases in the elderly's income. Therefore, the absence of adequate insurance coverage for prescription drugs may severely limit the elderly's ability to pay for necessary prescriptions. This is most likely to affect groups such as the elderly poor ineligible for Medicaid and the elderly poor living slightly above the poverty level—the groups least likely to have adequate drug insurance coverage.

Pharmaceutical companies, like most private enterprises, can be expected to continue to try to increase sales volume and average charge per prescription. Their motivation is to achieve profit margins considered to be "acceptable" by the industry. Current figures suggest that drug company profits per dollar of sale are high, relative to other industries. The Pharmaceutical Manufacturers Association reported that the industry's first-quarter profits per dollar of sale in 1986 were generated at an annual rate of 18.3 percent before taxes, well above the 5.7 percent for all manufacturing. After-tax profits for drugs were 12.6 percent, compared with 3.5 percent for all manufacturing (U.S. Bureau of the Census 1986).

Changes in Health Policy and Health Care Financing

In this book we reviewed the impact of federal regulation on the sale and use of prescription and nonprescription drugs. Two other areas of health policy are relevant: the government's support of biomedical, behavioral, and social sciences research, and its growing role in health care organization and financing. Although a complete discussion of these complex issues is beyond the scope of this book, we will highlight important trends that may have a significant impact on geriatric drug use. We recognize the hazards of fore-

* For example, use of cimetidine (Tagamet) for duodenal ulcer disease in a patient population spanning all ages led to an estimated 26 to 70 percent cost savings for Michigan's Medicaid program in the first year of use. In some cases, at least, these dramatic cost savings resulted from substituting Tagamet for duodenal ulcer surgery (Geweke & Weisbrod 1982).

casting future developments in health policy, but we will try to substantiate our predictions with the recent projections made by health professionals (Ginzberg 1985; Tyson & Merrill 1984; Blendon 1986).

Biomedical, Behavioral, and Social Sciences Research

In the past fifty years, dramatic progress has been made in the research and development of medical technologies. Progress has been fueled, first, by the federal government's financial support for biomedical research and research training. It has been fueled, too, by private industry's investments in research and development. Finally, technological advances have been made in academic health science centers, where the development of new drugs and devices is encouraged.

Some developments taking place in university laboratories, research institutes, and industry are likely to help reduce the costs of health care:

☐ Continued advances in molecular biology, genetics, pharmaceutical chemistry, and pharmacology are likely to provide drugs that are more effective and less likely to produce side effects.

☐ Computers and fiberoptic networking are producing medical and management information systems that permit more detailed monitoring of the practice patterns of physicians. Such information systems make possible improved systems of quality control and drug utilization review.

☐ New monitoring devices, advances in anesthesia and surgery, and new drugs will probably accelerate the trend toward ambulatory, rather than inpatient, hospital care.

At the same time, other devices, such as artificial implants and organ transplants, will probably become more common. These devices will do little to reduce costs, although they may prolong the lives of some patients and enhance the quality of life for many others.

Health Care Organization and Financing

Ever since health statistics have been maintained, care costs have been rising more rapidly than most other costs. In fact, since the late 1970s, rising costs have become the major policy issue in health care. National expenditures for health care have risen from 5.3 percent of gross national product (GNP) in 1960 to 7.6 percent in 1970 to 10.9 percent in 1986. National health care expenditures rose to $458 billion in 1986 and are expected to reach $660 billion in 1990 and $2 trillion by 2000 (14 percent of GNP). At this rate of increase, health care expenditures will double every seven years, and per capita spending will increase from $1,500 in 1984 to $7,000 in 2000

(Blendon 1986). These rising health care expenditures have led to efforts to contain health care costs.

One such initiative that could have significant implications not only for cost-containment but also for the elderly's drug use, spending, and quality of care has been the federal government's effort to enroll Medicare beneficiaries in competitive medical care plans (CMPs), such as health maintenance organizations, or HMOs,* and preferred provider organizations, or PPOs.† The Tax Equity and Fiscal Responsibility Act (TEFRA) of 1982 contains a provision authorizing HCFA to negotiate at-risk contracts‡ with such prepaid medical plans. The ability of HMOs to achieve cost savings through reduced hospitalization rates, the fiscal crisis confronting Medicare, and a desire to stimulate competition in the medical marketplace have made members of Congress receptive to proposals making these plans more available to Medicare beneficiaries (Luft 1981; Aiken & Bays 1984). The number of Medicare beneficiaries enrolled in HMOs has grown from 1.5 percent in 1981 to 5.4 percent in 1985 (Fingerhut & Rosenberg 1984; Interstudy 1986).

Proponents of competitive medical care plans argue that such plans offer elderly patients more benefits per Medicare dollar because of their organization and financing, which encourage tighter controls on hospital use, and their use of peer review of all services. Some prepaid medical plans also offer a variety of services in one location, thus enhancing accessibility of care. Furthermore, there is the potential for coordinating the services of specialists with those of primary care physicians and for monitoring use of multiple medications. Physicians in CMPs are more likely to have economic incentives to use generic drugs and may be more receptive to having pharmacists substitute less expensive drugs for equivalent brand-name products. If more of the elderly were enrolled in capitated prepaid health plans, there would probably be reductions both in the unnecessary utilization of drugs and in their costs.

On the other hand, these plans may have some potential disadvantages. Because they operate according to economic incentives that can encourage underuse of services (in contrast to fee-for-service systems that can encourage

---

*An HMO is an organization that provides comprehensive health services to an enrolled population for a fixed periodic payment.

†A PPO is an entity sponsored by health care providers (hospitals, physicians, and/or allied health professionals), by payers for health services (insurers, prepaid health systems, employers, and unions), and by third-party administrators or insurance brokers. Typically, providers in PPOs accept fixed rates of payment (often at levels below their regular charges) and agree to adhere to a utilization review program.

‡An "at-risk" contract is one in which the plan is paid an annual capitation rate equal to 95 percent of Medicare's adjusted average per capita cost (AAPCC) for the area—that is, 95 percent of the average cost in the plan's county for fee-for-service Medicare beneficiaries with characteristics similar to those of the plan's members.

overuse), there is a higher probability that some health problems of the elderly may be undiagnosed. Thus, some drugs which would be beneficial to the elderly may not be prescribed.

Competitive medical care plan enrollees will probably grow as a percentage of the total Medicare population. However, unless there is rapid growth in the development of these programs—and substantial participation by office-based physicians in them—it is unlikely that more than 20 percent of the Medicare enrollees will be enrolled in CMPs by 1990. The growth in enrollment in CMPs will probably result from the "aging in" of those currently enrolled in CMPs into the Medicare program, rather than from wholesale switching of the elderly from their usual physicians to ones affiliated with CMPs.

The Impact of Alternative Population Projections on Use, Price, and Spending for Prescription Drugs

The Authors and Mark S. Freeland

In this brief appendix we examine the effect of two alternative population projections on use, price, and spending for prescription drugs.

Alternative Population Projections to 2050

Population projections far into the future are based on explicit and implicit assumptions that may turn out to be erroneous. Consequently, Social Security actuaries develop three sets of projections. The baseline projections are the Alternative II, or Intermediate, projections. They correspond closely to the Census Bureau middle series projection and are considered the most accurate of the three sets (Wade 1985). The Intermediate set was the basis for the projections in Appendix A on use, price, and spending for prescription drugs.

Each of the three sets is based on a different set of assumptions for fertility rates, mortality rates, and net immigration (Table B.1). The Intermediate projections assume a fertility rate of 2.0 (that is, 2.0 births per woman), life expectancy of 76.4 for males and 84.0 for females, and a net annual immigration rate of 500,000 persons. Of the three sets of projections, Alternative I is designed to produce the most favorable financial impact on the Medicare and Social Security Trust Funds. In order to do so, these projections assume higher fertility rates, lower life expectancy, and higher net immigration. Each of these assumptions contributes to a lower proportion of aged persons to the total population and to a lower aged or gerontic dependency ratio (the ratio of aged persons to persons 20 to 64 years of age).

The Alternative III projections are structured to produce a less favorable impact on the Medicare and Social Security Trust Funds than are Alternative

TABLE B.I

Basic Assumptions Underlying the Three Projection Alternatives:
Fertility, Mortality, and Net Immigration

Projection alternative	Fertility: ultimate lifetime births per woman	Mortality: life expectancy at birth in 2050		Annual net immigration
		Male	Female	
Alternative II (Intermediate)	2.0	76.4	84.0	500,000
Alternative I	2.3	73.9	81.2	700,000
Alternative III	1.6	80.8	88.6	300,000

SOURCE: Wade 1985.

II projections. Thus, they assume lower fertility rates, higher life expectancy, and lower net immigration. Each of these assumptions results in a higher proportion of aged persons to the total population and to higher aged (gerontic) dependency ratios.

As can be expected from the assumptions in Table B.1, the Alternative I projections show the fastest total population growth. The population reaches 390 million by 2050, a 65 percent increase since 1980 (Table B.2). This is 19 percent higher than the population total of 327 million in the Alternative II projections (Appendix A, Table A.1).

The primary reason for the faster growth of total population in Alternative I is the higher fertility rate and the consequent faster growth of the nonaged population. The elderly are a lower proportion of total population for each projected year in the Alternative I projection than in Intermediate projections (Table B.4). Geronic dependency ratios are lower in the Alternative I projection, while neontic dependency ratios—ratios of persons under 20 years to persons 20 to 64 years of age—are higher (Table B.5).

Of the three sets, Alternative III has the slowest growth in total population, primarily because of lower fertility rates and the accompanying slower growth in the nonaged population. There is a decline in the nonaged population from 210 million in 1980 to 182 million in 2050 (Table B.3). The elderly progressively become a substantially higher proportion of the total population in the Alternative III projections (Table B.4). The gerontic dependency ratios are the highest for this scenario, and the neontic dependency ratios are the lowest (Table B.5). As a consequence of the cumulative more rapid percentage growth in the elderly, the absolute numbers of aged persons added each successive decade are higher in this scenario than in either of the other two scenarios (Table B.6).

TABLE B.2

Historical and Projected Population Figures, Alternative I, 1950–2050

Year	Total population		Population under 65		Population 65 and older	
	In thousands	Pct. change from previous decade	In thousands	Pct. change from previous decade	In thousands	Pct. change from previous decade
1950	157,313	+14.3%	144,712	+12.9%	12,601	+37.0%
1960	188,943	+20.2	171,797	+18.6	17,147	+35.9
1970	214,034	+13.2	193,351	+12.6	20,684	+20.6
1980	235,885	+10.3	209,784	+8.4	26,100	+26.3
1990	259,922	+10.2	227,714	+8.6	32,208	+23.4
2000	282,716	+8.8	247,482	+8.7	35,235	+9.4
2010	305,626	+8.1	266,352	+7.6	39,274	+11.5
2020	328,640	+7.6	277,131	+4.1	51,510	+31.1
2030	349,472	+6.3	285,223	+2.9	64,249	+24.8
2040	369,224	+5.6	303,397	+6.4	65,827	+2.4
2050	389,558	+5.5	323,647	+6.7	65,911	+0.1

SOURCE: Wade 1985.

TABLE B.3
Historical and Projected Population Figures, Alternative III, 1950–2050

Year	Total population		Population under 65		Population 65 and older	
	In thousands	Pct. change from previous decade	In thousands	Pct. change from previous decade	In thousands	Pct. change from previous decade
1950	157,313	+14.3%	144,712	+12.9%	12,601	+37.0%
1960	188,943	+20.2	171,797	+18.6	17,147	+35.9
1970	214,034	+13.2	193,351	+12.6	20,684	+20.6
1980	235,885	+10.3	209,784	+8.4	26,100	+26.3
1990	256,345	+8.7	223,670	+7.7	32,675	+25.2
2000	270,023	+5.3	232,450	+6.6	37,573	+15.0
2010	278,955	+3.4	235,325	+3.9	43,629	+16.1
2020	283,317	+1.6	224,975	+1.2	58,342	+33.7
2030	281,798	−0.6	207,444	−4.3	74,354	+27.5
2040	274,915	−2.4	195,667	−7.8	79,248	+6.6
2050	263,420	−4.3	181,786	−5.7	81,634	+3.0

SOURCE: Wade 1985.

TABLE B.4

*Percent of Historical and Projected Total Population 65 and Over,
by Projection Alternative, 1950–2050*

Year	Alternative II (Intermediate)	Alternative I	Alternative III
1950	8.0%		
1960	9.1		
1970	9.7		
1980	11.1		
1990	12.6	12.4%	12.7%
2000	13.2	12.5	13.9
2010	14.1	12.9	15.6
2020	17.7	15.9	20.6
2030	21.5	18.4	26.4
2040	21.9	17.8	28.8
2050	21.8	16.9	31.0

SOURCE: Wade 1985.

Projecting Use, Price, and Spending for Prescription Drugs: The Historical Data Base and the Computational Method

The Historical Data Base

The historical data base used for estimating prescriptions per capita, charges per prescription, and charges per capita (the number of prescriptions per capita multiplied by the average charge per prescription) by age and sex is made up of unpublished tabulations from the National Center for Health Services Research National Medical Care Expenditures Survey (NMCES). Of the two most current and relevant data sources, the 1977 NMCES and the 1980 Health Care Financing Administration/National Center for Health Statistics National Medical Care Utilization and Expenditure Survey (NMCUES), the NMCES survey seemed most appropriate for our purposes. Both surveys are of households in the civilian noninstitutionalized population. However, the NMCES survey was supplemented by additional surveys of physicians and health care facilities providing care to household members and of insurance companies and employers responsible for insurance coverage of the households (Kasper 1982). The increased reliability associated with the supplemental NMCES surveys seemed to more than compensate for potential changes in use and charge relationships between 1977 and 1980.

TABLE B.5
Historical and Projected Societal Dependency Ratios, by Projection Alternative, 1950–2050

	Societal dependency ratios								
	Alternative II (Intermediate)			Alternative I			Alternative III		
Year	Total	Neontic	Gerontic	Total	Neontic	Gerontic	Total	Neontic	Gerontic
1950	72.1	58.3	13.8						
1960	91.5	74.1	17.4						
1970	90.1	71.7	18.4						
1980	74.9	55.5	19.4						
1990	69.2	47.9	21.3	63.3	48.3	21.0	68.9	47.4	21.5
2000	67.2	45.2	22.0	68.5	47.5	21.0	65.0	42.0	23.0
2010	64.9	41.7	23.2	68.0	46.4	21.6	60.4	35.3	25.1
2020	73.7	43.0	30.7	77.1	49.3	27.8	69.2	34.4	34.8
2030	84.3	44.7	39.6	86.6	52.3	34.3	82.6	34.4	48.2
2040	84.8	44.3	40.5	85.6	52.5	33.1	87.3	33.3	54.0
2050	85.0	44.6	40.4	84.1	53.0	31.1	93.5	33.5	60.0

SOURCE: Wade 1985.

NOTE: The terminology for dependency ratios is from Siegel and Taeuber 1986. The ratios are constructed as follows. "Total" ratios are an expression of the population under 20 plus the population 65 and over divided by the population 20 to 64, times 100. "Neontic" ratios are an expression of the population under 20 divided by the population 20 to 64, times 100. "Gerontic" ratios are an expression of the population 65 and over divided by the population 20 to 64, times 100.

TABLE B.6

Population 65 and Over, and Increases from Previous Decade, by Projection Alternative, 1950–2050

Year	Alternative II (Intermediate) Pop. 65 and over (000)	Increase from previous decade No. (000)	Pct.	Alternative I Pop. 65 and over (000)	Increase from previous decade No. (000)	Pct.	Alternative III Pop. 65 and over (000)	Increase from previous decade No. (000)	Pct.
1950	12,601	3,407	+37.0%						
1960	17,147	4,546	+35.9						
1970	20,684	3,537	+20.6						
1980	26,100	5,416	+26.3						
1990	32,448	6,348	+24.3	32,208	6,108	+23.4%	32,675	6,575	+25.2%
2000	36,445	3,997	+12.3	35,235	3,027	+9.4	37,573	4,898	+15.0
2010	41,362	4,917	+13.5	39,274	4,039	+11.5	43,629	6,056	+16.1
2020	54,484	13,122	+31.7	51,510	12,236	+31.1	58,342	14,713	+33.7
2030	68,280	13,796	+25.3	64,249	12,739	+24.8	74,354	16,012	+27.5
2040	70,791	2,511	+3.7	65,827	1,578	+2.4	79,248	4,894	+6.6
2050	71,340	549	+0.8	65,911	84	+0.1	81,634	2,386	+3.0

SOURCE: Wade 1985.

To examine the sensitivity of the analysis to the use of the NMCUES data rather than the NMCES data, analysis was done using both data bases. Prescriptions per capita, charges per prescription, and charges per capita by age and sex were projected forward to 2050 and backward to 1950, using the two independent sets of use and charge rates. Whereas the estimated levels of prescriptions per capita, charges per prescription, and charges per capita by age and sex differed for the 1980 NMCUES survey compared with the 1977 NMCES survey, the two data sources produced essentially identical effects for the aging of the population. This reflects the fact that *relative* use and charge rates for the various age-sex groups are approximately the same for the two surveys.

Estimates of prescriptions per capita, charges per prescription and charges per capita by five-year age intervals are shown in Table B.7.* The number of prescriptions per capita for males and females rises steadily from the teenage years and reaches a plateau at approximately age 75 to 84, then tends to decline. This decline may, in part, reflect the fact that the household survey is for the noninstitutionalized population only. Elderly persons who suffer the greatest morbidity and use the most prescription drugs may be institutionalized, especially in nursing homes. However, some data sources for other services, such as hospital care, include the institutionalized population. These sources also show lower utilization rates for people approximately age 85 years and older (Arnett, McKusick, Sonnefeld & Cowell 1986). Perhaps persons who survive to this very old age are on average a select (this is, healthier) population. (See Chapter 2 for detailed analyses of factors contributing to differential use of prescription drugs by age and gender.)

Average charge per prescription tends to rise slowly but steadily with age for both males and females. On average, males pay slightly higher charges per prescription than do females. Average charge per capita (the number of prescriptions per capita multiplied by the average charge per prescription) tends to follow the pattern of average number of prescriptions per capita, because there is relatively little variation in the average charge per prescription by age and sex compared with the average number of prescriptions per capita by age and sex (Table B.7).

The Computation Method

The computation method used to project changes in average use and charge rates caused solely by changes in the age-sex composition of the population is standard and follows the same procedure as Arnett, McKusick,

---

* An actuarial smoothing technique, the Whittaker-Henderson type B graduation procedure (Miller 1946), was used to reduce the effect of sampling variability associated with the relatively small number of observations for some of the age categories.

TABLE B.7

Number of Prescriptions Per Capita, Average Charge Per Prescription, and
Average Charges Per Capita, by Age and Sex, 1977

Age category	No. of prescriptions per capita		Ave. charge per prescription		Ave. charges per capita	
	Females	Males	Females	Males	Females	Males
0–4	2.1	2.9	$4.78	$4.85	$9.87	$13.77
5–9	2.0	2.2	4.97	4.99	9.65	11.19
10–14	2.0	1.7	5.11	5.11	10.33	8.96
15–19	2.5	1.4	5.23	5.22	12.82	7.83
20–24	3.1	1.4	5.33	5.33	16.46	7.85
25–29	3.8	1.5	5.44	5.47	20.09	9.01
30–34	4.3	1.9	5.54	5.65	23.59	11.64
35–39	4.9	2.5	5.65	5.92	27.87	15.91
40–44	5.7	3.2	5.82	6.17	34.05	21.24
45–49	6.7	4.0	6.01	6.43	41.54	27.07
50–54	7.9	5.0	6.18	6.63	49.67	33.52
55–59	9.1	6.1	6.29	6.80	57.86	41.10
60–64	10.3	7.2	6.37	6.92	65.76	48.76
65–69	11.3	8.2	6.44	7.02	72.58	55.12
70–74	12.2	8.8	6.47	7.11	78.20	58.90
75–79	12.8	9.1	6.47	7.17	82.15	60.67
80–84	13.0	9.1	6.48	7.10	82.65	59.88
85–89	12.4	8.7	6.48	6.70	77.28	55.64
90–94	10.8	7.3	6.60	6.17	65.38	45.79
95+	8.1	5.4	6.90	5.56	48.47	32.49

SOURCE: Unpublished tabulations from NCHSR National Health Care Expenditures Study.
NOTE: See Kasper (1982) for background of study relating to prescribed medicines. The
tabulations were smoothed, using the Whittaker-Henderson type B graduation procedure
(Miller 1946). Average charges per capita distributions for males and females were smoothed
independently from the number of prescriptions per capita and average charge per prescription
distributions in order to obtain the best Whittaker-Henderson fit for the average charges per
capita distributions.

Sonnefeld, and Cowell (1986), Davis and Rowland (1986), and Russell
(1981). The use or charge rates for each age-sex category in Table B.7 were
multiplied by the number of persons in those same age-sex categories (Wade
1985) to derive total use or charges for persons in the specific age-sex categories.* Use or charges were added up for the aged, nonaged, and total popula-

* In the case of average charge per prescription, an additional computation was
necessary. Average charges per prescription within age-sex categories were multiplied
by total number of prescriptions within the respective age-sex categories to properly
weigh the average charges per prescription across age-sex categories.

tions to obtain aggregate use and charges for these three population groups. The use and charge aggregates for the three population groups were then divided by the total population of each of the groups to calculate use and charge rates for different years from 1950 to 2050. Per capita number of prescriptions, average charge per prescription, and average charge per capita for the aged, nonaged, and total populations change from year to year as the proportions of persons in the various age-sex categories change.

The computation method holds constant the per capita number of prescriptions, the average charge per prescription, and the average charge per capita *within* each of the forty age-sex categories—the twenty age categories each for females and for males—in Table B.7. Changes in the age-sex composition of the population are the only reason for per capita number of prescriptions, average charge per prescription, and average charge per capita for the aged, nonaged, and total populations changing from one year to another. By holding constant all factors except age-sex composition and population size, we can determine the effects of these population changes on use, price, and spending for prescription drugs.

The computation method was applied to the historical estimates of the population and to each of the three population projections made by Social Security actuaries (Wade 1985). The projections of number of persons by age to 2050 for the three alternatives are shown in Tables A.1, B.2, and B.3. Projections of use, price, per capita charges, and total charges for the three scenarios are shown in Tables B.10, B.11, and B.12.

TABLE B.8

Number of Prescriptions, Total Index and Per Capita, for the Nonaged (Under 65) Population, Alternative II (Intermediate), 1950–2050

	No. of prescriptions			
Year	Total index (1977 = 100)	Pct. change from previous decade	Per capita	Pct. change from previous decade
1950	71.6	+15.7%	3.6	+2.6%
1960	83.9	+17.3	3.6	−1.4
1970	94.1	+12.1	3.6	−0.3
1980	103.2	+9.7	3.6	+1.1
1990	113.1	+9.5	3.7	+1.7
2000	127.0	+12.4	3.9	+5.5
2010	141.5	+11.4	4.1	+6.2
2020	143.0	+1.1	4.1	+0.7
2030	136.8	−4.3	4.0	−2.7
2040	138.9	+1.5	4.0	0.0
2050	140.5	+1.2	4.0	0.0

TABLE B.9

Total Index, Per Capita, and Per Prescription Index Charges for Prescription Drugs for the Nonaged (Under 65) Population, Alternative II (Intermediate), 1950–2050

Year	Total index (1977 = 100)	Pct. change from previous decade	Charges for prescription drugs (constant 1977 dollars)				
			Per capita	Pct. change from previous decade	Per prescription index (1977 = 100)	Pct. change from previous decade	
1950	71.4	+15.5%	$21.29	+2.5%	99.7	+0.1%
1960	83.5	+16.9	20.97	−1.5	99.5	−0.2
1970	93.9	+12.5	20.95	−0.1	99.8	+0.3
1980	103.3	+10.0	21.23	+1.3	100.0	+0.2
1990	113.4	+9.8	21.66	+2.0	100.0	+0.1
2000	128.9	+13.7	23.11	+6.7	101.2	+1.1
2010	145.0	+12.5	24.79	+7.3	102.4	+1.2
2020	146.6	+1.1	24.97	+0.7	102.6	+0.2
2030	139.7	−4.7	24.19	−3.1	102.0	−0.6
2040	141.8	+1.5	24.22	+0.1	102.1	+0.1
2050	143.5	+1.2	24.23	0.0	102.1	0.0

Number of Prescriptions Per Capita, by Projection Alternative, 1950–2050

Year	Alternative II (Intermediate)			Alternative I			Alternative III		
	Total	Under 65	65 and older	Total	Under 65	65 and older	Total	Under 65	65 and older
1950	4.2	3.5	10.4	4.2	3.5	10.4	4.2	3.5	10.4
1970	4.2	3.6	10.7	4.2	3.6	10.7	4.2	3.6	10.7
1990	4.5	3.7	10.7	4.5	3.6	10.7	4.6	3.7	10.7
2010	5.0	4.1	10.6	4.9	4.0	10.6	5.2	4.2	10.6
2030	5.4	4.0	10.6	5.1	3.8	10.6	5.9	4.3	10.5
2050	5.4	4.0	10.5	5.0	3.8	10.6	6.2	4.4	10.3

TABLE B.11

Index of Average Charges Per Prescription, by Projection Alternative, 1950–2050
(1977 = 100)

Year	Alternative II (Intermediate)			Alternative I			Alternative III		
	Total	Under 65	65 and older	Total	Under 65	65 and older	Total	Under 65	65 and older
1950	99.1	99.7	100.6	99.1	99.7	100.6	99.1	99.7	100.6
1970	99.6	99.8	100.1	99.6	99.8	100.1	99.6	99.8	100.1
1990	100.5	100.1	100.0	100.4	100.0	100.0	100.6	100.2	100.0
2010	102.1	102.4	100.1	101.6	102.0	100.0	102.7	102.9	100.1
2030	103.4	102.0	100.3	102.5	101.2	100.2	104.6	103.2	100.3
2050	103.3	102.1	101.1	102.0	101.1	101.1	105.1	103.6	100.0

TABLE B.12

Average Charges Per Capita for Prescription Drugs, by Projection Alternative, 1950–2050
(1977 Dollars)

Year	Alternative II (Intermediate)			Alternative I			Alternative III		
	Total	Under 65	65 and older	Total	Under 65	65 and older	Total	Under 65	65 and older
1950	$25.02	$21.29	$67.85	$25.02	$21.29	$67.85	$25.02	$21.29	$67.85
1970	25.61	20.95	69.15	25.61	20.95	69.15	25.61	20.95	69.15
1990	27.63	21.66	69.21	27.51	21.61	69.23	27.77	21.72	69.20
2010	30.94	24.79	68.46	29.92	24.20	68.70	32.27	25.62	68.18
2030	33.71	24.19	68.46	31.42	23.01	68.77	37.17	26.11	68.01
2050	33.69	24.23	67.60	30.49	22.80	68.24	39.02	26.68	66.49

TABLE B.13

Index of Total Charges for Prescribed Medicines, by Projection Alternative, 1950–2050
(1977 = 100)

Year	Alternative II (Intermediate)			Alternative I			Alternative III		
	Total	Under 65	65 and older	Total	Under 65	65 and older	Total	Under 65	65 and older
1950	65.6	71.4	50.7	65.6	71.4	50.7	65.6	71.4	50.7
1970	91.4	93.9	84.9	91.4	93.9	84.9	91.4	93.9	84.9
1990	119.0	113.4	133.3	119.2	114.1	132.3	118.7	112.7	134.2
2010	151.5	145.0	168.0	152.4	149.4	160.1	150.1	139.8	176.5
2030	178.4	139.7	277.4	183.0	152.1	262.1	174.6	125.6	300.0
2050	183.6	143.5	286.2	198.0	171.1	266.9	171.3	112.4	322.1

Results for Alternative Projections

It is interesting to compare and contrast Alternative I and III projections of use, charges per prescription, and charges per capita to 2050 with the Intermediate projections. The major difference in the three projections of population is in the absolute size of the nonaged population. In the Intermediate projection, the projected number of nonaged persons in 2050 is 255 million (Table A.1). This number is 41 percent higher than the 182 million projected in Alternative III (Table B.3). In contrast, Alternative I, in which 324 million nonaged persons are projected for 2050, yields a number 27 percent higher than does the Intermediate projection.

The relatively rapid growth in the nonaged population in the Alternative I projection translates into a faster rate of growth in total prescriptions for the nonaged compared with growth in Alternative II. Similarly, the slower growth in the nonaged population in Alternative III is associated with slower growth in total prescriptions compared with Alternative II.

The longer life expectancy assumed in Alternative III (Table B.1) results in faster growth of the elderly population (Table B.6) compared with the Alternative II projections. This, in turn, results in faster growth in total number of prescriptions for the elderly and a faster rate of increase in per capita number of prescriptions for the total population (Table B.10).

Average charges per prescription for the total and nonaged populations rise fastest for Alternative III and slowest for Alternative I (Table B.11). Average charge per prescription for the elderly population is essentially unaffected in the three scenarios, because the average charge per prescription is relatively flat when males and females are averaged together (Table B.7).

Average charge per capita for the elderly shows little variation among the three scenarios (Table B.12) because of the parabolic shape (increase, then plateau, then decrease) of the underlying distribution of per capita charges (Table B.7). For the nonaged and total populations, Alternative III shows the greatest increase in charges per capita, and Alternative I the least increase in charges per capita from 1950 to 2050.

Projections of total charges reflect the impact of changes in the size of the population on number of prescriptions and changes in the age-sex composition of the population on number of prescriptions per capita and average charge per prescription (Table B.10, Table B.11). The index of total charges for prescription drugs for total population in Alternative I reaches 198 in 2050, double the 1977 base of 100.0 but only 8 percent higher than for Alternative II, in which the index is 183.6 (Table B.13). This reflects the fact that Alternative I total population is 19 percent higher than Alternative II total population in 2050, but Alternative I has lower projected average number of prescriptions per capita (Table B.10). As shown in Table B.11, Alter-

TABLE B.14

Average Annual Rates of Change for Total Prescriptions, Population, and Age-Sex Index of Prescription Drug Use Per Capita, Selected Periods, 1970–85

	1970–75	1975–80	1980–85	1970–80	1970–85
Total Prescriptions[a]	+3.1%	−1.3%	+2.1%	+0.9%	+1.3%
Total Population	+1.0	+1.0	+1.0	+1.0	+1.0
No. of prescriptions per capita[b]	+2.1	−2.3	+1.2	−0.1	+0.3
Age-sex index of prescription drug use per capita[c]	+0.3	+0.4	+0.3	+0.3	+0.3
No. of prescriptions per capita deflated by the age-sex index of prescriptions per capita[d]	+1.8	−2.6	+0.8	−0.4	0.0

SOURCES: IMS America, Ltd.; Wade 1985.

[a]Total prescriptions are usually reported in the April issue of *Pharmacy Times*.

[b]Total prescriptions divided by total population. Note that the Social Security Area Population includes some persons not included in the IMS America, Ltd. data base. This results in a slightly lower per capita number of prescriptions, but the trend in number of prescriptions should not be significantly affected.

[c]Division of National Cost Estimates, Office of the Actuary, Health Care Financing Administration, Baltimore, Md., unpublished. Also see Table A.3 in Appendix A.

[d]This series reflects the number of prescriptions per capita after effects of age and sex have been factored out.

TABLE B.15

Average Annual Rates of Change for Average Charge Per Prescription, Consumer Price Index for Prescription Drugs, and Age-Sex Index of Average Charge Per Prescription, Selected Periods, 1970–85

	1970–75	1975–80	1980–85	1970–80	1970–85
Ave. charge per prescription[a]	+5.3%	+8.1%	+11.3%	+6.7%	+8.2%
CPI for Prescription Drugs	+1.6	+7.2	+10.6	+4.3	+6.4
Deflated ave. charge per prescription[b]	+3.7	+0.8	+ 0.6	+2.2	+1.7
Age-sex index of ave. charge per prescription[c]	+0.1	+0.1	0.0	+0.1	+0.1
Residual deflated charge per prescription[d]	+3.6	+0.7	+ 0.6	+2.2	+1.7

SOURCES: IMS America, Ltd.; Bureau of Labor Statistics.

[a] Average charge per prescription is usually reported in the April issue of *Pharmacy Times*.

[b] Average charge per prescription deflated by the Consumer Price Index for Prescription Drugs.

[c] Division of National Cost Estimates, Office of the Actuary, Health Care Financing Administration, Baltimore, Md., unpublished. See also Table A.5 in Appendix A.

[d] Deflated average charge per prescription deflated by the age-sex index of average charge per prescription.

native I also has lower average charge per prescription than does Alternative II, because Alternative I has, on average, a younger population.

The projected index of total charges for Alternative III for total population is 171.3 in 2050 compared with 183.6 for Alternative II, or 7 percent less (Table B.13). Total population is 19 percent less for Alternative III in 2050. However, both average number of prescriptions per capita (Table B.10) and average charge per prescription are higher for Alternative III compared with Alternative II, because Alternative III has an older population.

A major conclusion from this analysis of alternative population projections is that population growth shows more variability than does growth in total charges for prescription drugs. This is so because rapid growth in total population is associated with a younger population and, thus, fewer prescriptions per capita and lower average charge per prescription. Similarly, slower growth in total population is associated with an older population and concomitant higher average number of prescriptions per capita and higher average charge per prescription.

Bibliography

Aiken, L. H., and K. D. Bays. 1984. The Medicare debate—Round one. *New England Journal of Medicine* 311: 1196–1200.

Alderman, M. H., and E. E. Schoenbaum. 1975. Detection and treatment of hypertension in the work site. *New England Journal of Medicine* 293: 65–67.

Alonzo, A. A. 1979. Everyday illness behavior: A situational approach to health status deviations. *Social Science and Medicine* 13A: 397–404.

Amenn, G. S. 1982. Pharmacogenetics. In *Annual Review of Gerontology and Geriatrics*, ed. C. Eisdorfer, pp. 27–51. New York: Springer. Vol. 3.

American Association of Colleges of Pharmacy and Eli Lilly and Company. 1985. *Pharmacy practice for the geriatric patient.* Carrboro, N.C.: Health Sciences Consortium.

American Association of Retired Persons. 1984. *Prescription drugs: A survey of consumer use, attitudes, and behavior.* Washington, D.C.

———. 1985. *Cuts in social security cost-of-living adjustments (COLAS): Impact analysis.* Mimeo.

———. 1987. Testimony before the U.S. House Subcommittee on Health and the Environment, Energy and Commerce Committee. Washington, D.C., Apr. 21, 1987.

American Pharmaceutical Association. 1982. *Report of the policy committee on professional affairs.* Washington, D.C.

Andersen, R. 1968. *Model of families' use of health services.* Chicago, Ill.: Center for Health Services Administration Studies, Research Series No. 25.

Andersen, R., B. Smedby, and A. Anderson. 1970. *Medical care use in Sweden and the United States—A comparative analysis of systems and behavior.* Chicago, Ill.: Center for Health Services Administration Studies, Research Series No. 27.

Armstrong, W. A., Jr., C. W. Driever, and R. L. Hays. 1980. Analysis of drug-drug interactions in a geriatric population. *American Journal of Hospital Pharmacy* 37: 385–87.

Arnett, R. H., III, D. R. McKusick, S. T. Sonnefeld, and C. S. Cowell.

1986. Projections of health care spending to 1990. *Health Care Financing Review* 7, Spring 1986, pp. 1–36.

Arnett, R. H., III, et al. 1985. Health spending trends in the 1980s: Adjusting to financial incentives. *Health Care Financing Review* 6, Spring 1985, pp. 1–26.

Avorn, J. 1983. Drug policy in the aging society. *Health Affairs* 2: 23–32.

———. 1984. Benefit and cost analysis in geriatric care: Turning age discrimination into health policy. *New England Journal of Medicine* 310: 1294–1300.

Avorn, J., and S. B. Soumerai. 1982. Use of computer-based Medicaid drug data to analyze and correct inappropriate medication use. *Journal of Medical Systems* 6: 377–86.

———. 1983. Improving drug-therapy decisions through educational outreach: A randomized controlled trial of academically based "detailing." *New England Journal of Medicine* 308: 1457–63.

Avorn, J., M. Chen, and R. Hartley. 1982. Scientific versus commercial sources of influence on the prescribing behavior of physicians. *American Journal of Medicine* 73: 4–8.

Balint, M. 1964. *The doctor, his patient, and the illness.* London: Pitman.

Balter, M. B., and M. L. Bauer. 1975. Patterns of prescribing and use of hypnotic drugs in the United States. Chap. 12 in *Sleep disturbance and hypnotic drug dependence*, ed. A. Clift. Amsterdam: Excerpta Medica.

Balter, M. B., J. Levine, and D. Manheimer. 1974. Cross-national study of the extent of anti-anxiety/sedative drug use. *New England Journal of Medicine* 290: 769–74.

Basen, M. 1977. The elderly and drugs: Problems, overview, and program strategy. *Public Health Reports* 92: 38–43.

Baum, C., D. L. Kennedy, and M. B. Forbes. 1985. Drug utilization in the geriatric age group. In *Geriatric drug use—Clinical and social perspectives*, eds. S. R. Moore and T. W. Teal, pp. 63–69. New York: Pergamon.

Baum, C., D. L. Kennedy, M. B. Forbes, and J. K. Jones. 1985. Drug use and expenditures in 1982. *Journal of the American Medical Association* 253: 382–83.

Baum, C., et al. 1984. Drug use in the United States in 1981. *Journal of the American Medical Association* 251: 1293–97.

Beck, J. C., et al. 1982. Dementia in the elderly: The silent epidemic. *Annals of Internal Medicine* 97: 231–41.

Becker, P. M., and H. J. Cohen. 1984. The functional approach to the care of the elderly: A conceptual framework. *Journal of the American Geriatrics Society* 32: 923–29.

Becker, P. M., R. Drachman, and J. Kirscht. 1972. Predicting mothers' compliance with pediatric medical regimens. *Pediatrics* 81: 843–54.

Becker, P. M., et al. 1971. Characteristics and attitudes of physicians associated with the prescribing of chloramphenicol. *HSMHA Health Reports* 86: 993–1003.

Beebe, K., W. Callahan, and A. Mariano. 1986. Medicare short-stay hospital length of stay, fiscal years 1981–1985. *Health Care Financing Review* 7, Spring 1986, pp. 119–25.

Bender, A. D. 1965. The effect of increasing age on the distribution of peripheral blood flow in man. *Journal of the American Geriatrics Society* 13: 192–98.

Bergman, A., and R. Werner. 1963. Failure of children to receive penicillin by mouth. *New England Journal of Medicine* 268: 1334–38.

Bergman, U., and B. E. Wiholm. 1981. Drug-related problems causing admission to a medical clinic. *European Journal of Clinical Pharmacology* 20: 193–200.

Berkman, L. F., and L. Syme. 1979. Social networks, host resistance, and mortality. A nine-year follow-up study of Alameda County residents. *American Journal of Epidemiology* 109: 186–204.

Bezold, C. 1981. *The future of pharmaceuticals.* New York: Wiley.

Bezold, C., et al. 1984. *Pharmacy in the 21st century.* Washington, D.C.: Institute for Alternative Futures/Project Hope.

Blackwell, B. 1973. Drug therapy: Patient compliance. *New England Journal of Medicine* 289: 249–52.

Blaschke, T. F., et al. 1981. Drug-drug interactions and aging. In *Pharmacology of the aged*, eds. D. J. Greenblatt and L. F. Jarvic, pp. 11–26. New York: Raven.

Blendon, R. J. 1986. Health policy choices for the 1990s. *Issues in Science and Technology* 2: 65–73.

Blum, R., and K. Kreitman. 1981. Factors affecting individual use of medicine. In *Pharmaceuticals and health policy*, eds. R. Blum et al., pp. 122–85. London: Croom Helm.

Bonanno, J. B., and S. Wetle. 1984. HMO enrollment of Medicare recipients: An analysis of incentives and barriers. *Journal of Health Politics, Policy, and Law* 19: 41–62.

Bootzin, R. R., and M. Engle-Friedman. 1987. Sleep disturbances. In *Handbook of clinical gerontology*, eds. L. Carstensen and B. Edelstein, pp. 238–251. New York: Pergamon.

Boston Collaborative Drug Surveillance Program. 1973. Clinical depression of the central nervous system due to diazepam and chlordiazepoxide in relation to cigarette smoking and age. *New England Journal of Medicine* 288: 277–80.

Brand, F., and R. Smith. 1974. Medical care and compliance among the elderly after hospitalization. *International Journal of Aging and Human Development* 5: 331–46.

Brand, F. N., R. T. Smith, and P. A. Brand. 1977. Effect of economic barriers to medical care on patients' noncompliance. *Public Health Reports* 92: 72–78.

Braunstein, M. L., and J. D. James. 1976. A computer-based system for screening outpatient drug utilization. *Journal of the American Pharmaceutical Association* 16: 82–85.

Breitman, J. A. 1986. The pharmaceutical industry: Development and marketing of prescription drugs. In *Topics in clinical pharmacology and therapeutics*, ed. R. F. Maronde, pp. 500–509. New York: Springer-Verlag.

Brickfield, C. F. 1986. Pharmaceutical industry and the consumer: Renewing the trust. Presentation at a Conference on Pharmaceuticals for the Elderly: New Research and New Concerns. Washington, D.C., Feb. 13, 1986.

Brocklehurst, J. C., et al. 1978. Medical screening of old people accepted for residential care. *Lancet* 1: 141–42.

Brody, H., and D. S. Sobel. 1979. A systems view of health and disease. In *Ways of health*, ed. D. S. Sobel, pp. 87–104. New York: Harcourt Brace Jovanovich.

Brooks, P. M., et al. 1977. Reducing the pill swill: An audit of clinical pharmacy. *Medical Journal of Australia* 2: 427–28.

Brown, N. K., and D. J. Thompson. 1979. Non-treatment of fever in extended-care facilities. *New England Journal of Medicine* 300: 1246–50.

Bush, P. J., and D. L. Rabin. 1976. Who's using nonprescribed medicine? *Medical Care* 14: 1014–23.

———. 1977. Medicines: Who's using them? *Journal of the American Pharmaceutical Association* 14: 227–30.

Bush, P. J., and M. Osterweis. 1978. Pathways to medicine use. *Journal of Health and Social Behavior* 19: 179–89.

Butler, R. N. 1975. *Why survive? Being old in America*. New York: Harper & Row.

Butler, R. N., and M. I. Lewis. 1977. *Aging and mental health*. St. Louis, Mo.: C. V. Mosby.

Cabana, B. E. 1983. Mental health and the elderly: New biopharmaceutic considerations. *Health Affairs* 2: 33–38.

Califano, J. A. 1981. *Governing America. An insider's report from the White House and the Cabinet*. New York: Simon and Schuster.

California Assembly Bill 717. 1977. *An act to amend numerous sections and repeal numerous sections of the business and professional code and to amend numerous sections of the health and safety code relating to experimental health manpower projects*. Mar. 2, 1977 (Chapter 843 of California Statutes, Sept. 15, 1977).

California Assembly Bill 1868. 1981. Berman, Howard L. *An act to amend section 404b of the business and professions code, relating to pharmacy*. Sacramento, Mar. 30, 1981.

California Office of Statewide Health Planning and Development, Division of Health Professions Development. 1982. *Health manpower pilot projects:*

Annual report to the legislature, State of California and to the healing acts licensing boards. Nov. 1982.

Campion, E. W., et al. 1985. Age, weight, and dose in drug prescribing for ambulatory elders. Paper presented at the Gerontological Society of America Meeting, San Antonio, Texas, Nov. 22–26, 1985 (abstract).

Canada, A. T. 1976. The pharmacist and drug compliance. In *Compliance with therapeutic regimens*, eds. D. L. Sackett and R. D. Haynes. Baltimore, Md.: Johns Hopkins University Press.

Caplan, R. D., et al. 1976. *Adhering to medical regimens: Pilot experiments in patient education and social support.* Ann Arbor, Mich.: Institute for Social Research of the University of Michigan.

Caranasos, G. J., R. B. Stewart, and L. E. Cluff. 1974. Drug-induced illness leading to hospitalization. *Journal of the American Medical Association* 288: 713–17.

Castle, M., et al. 1977. Antibiotic use at Duke University Medical Center. *Journal of the American Medical Association* 237: 2819–33.

Center for Law and Social Policy. 1975. Petition to the FDA to require more adequate labeling of prescription drugs. Washington, D.C., 1975.

Chaiton, A., et al. 1976. Patterns of medical drug use—A community focus. *Canadian Medical Association Journal* 114: 33–37.

Charney, E., et al. 1967. How well do patients take oral penicillin? *Pediatrics* 40: 188–95.

Cheung, A., and R. Kayne. 1975. An application of clinical pharmacy services in extended care facilities. *California Pharmacist* 23: 22–28.

Cheung, A., et al. 1975. A prospective study of drug preparation and administration in extended care facilities. An unpublished study for U.S. Senate, Special Committee on Aging, Subcommittee on Long-Term Care, *Nursing home care in the United States: Failure in public policy. Supporting Paper No. 2, Drugs in nursing homes: Misuse, costs and kickbacks*, p. 279. Washington, D.C.: Government Printing Office.

Christakis, G., and A. Miridjanian. 1958. Diet, drugs, and their relationship. *Journal of the American Dietetic Association* 52: 22.

Closson, R. G., and C. A. Kikugawa. 1975. Noncompliance varies with drug class. *Hospitals* 49: 89–93.

Cluff, L. E. 1980. Is drug toxicity a problem of great magnitude? Yes! In *Controversies in therapeutics*, ed. L. Lasagna, pp. 44–50. Philadelphia: W. B. Saunders.

Coalition on Women and the Budget. 1983. *Inequality and sacrifice: The impact of the Reagan budget on women.* Washington, D.C.: National Women's Law Center.

Coates, T. J., and C. E. Thoresen. 1982. Treating sleep disorders: Few answers, some suggestions, and many questions. In *Handbook of clinical behavior therapy*, eds. S. M. Turner, K. S. Calhoun, and H. E. Adams. New York: Wiley.

Cohen, S. N., et al. 1974. Computer-based monitoring and reporting of drug interactions. *Proceedings of the International Federation of Information Processing Societies, Medical Information Conference*, pp. 689–94.

Cole, P., and S. Emmanuel. 1971. Drug consultation: Its significance to the discharged hospital patient and its relevance as a role for the pharmacist. *American Journal of Hospital Pharmacy* 28: 954–60.

Comanor, W. S. 1986. The political economy of the pharmaceutical industry. *Journal of Economic Literature* 24: 1187–1217.

Commission on the Federal Drug Approval Process. 1982. *Final report.* Washington, D.C.: Commission on the Federal Drug Approval Process, Apr. 23, 1982.

Conrad, K. A., and R. Bressler, eds. 1982. *Drug therapy for the elderly.* St. Louis, Mo.: C. V. Mosby.

Cooper, J. 1976. Food-drug interactions. *U.S. Pharmacist* 1: 13–28.

Cooper, J. K., D. W. Love, and P. R. Raffoul. 1982. Intentional prescription nonadherence (noncompliance) by the elderly. *Journal of the American Geriatrics Society* 30: 329–33.

Cooper, J. R., ed. 1978. Sedative-hypnotic drugs: Risks and benefits. DHHS Pub. No. (ADM) 81–592. U.S. Department of Health and Human Services, National Center for Health Services Research.

Cooper, J. W. 1978. Drug therapy in the elderly: Is it all it could be? *American Pharmacy* NS18: 25–26.

———. 1981. Pharmacology: Drug-related problems and the elderly. In *Eldercare: A practical guide to clinical geriatrics*, eds. M. O'Hara-Devereaux, L. H. Andrus, and C. D. Scott, pp. 65–81. New York: Grune and Stratton.

Cornoni-Huntley, J., and J. A. Brody. 1982. Established populations for epidemiologic studies of the elderly. Paper presented to 110th Annual American Public Health Association meeting, Montreal, Nov. 16, 1982.

Covington, T. R. 1983. Toward a rational approach to the issue of prescribing authority for pharmacists. *Drug Intelligence and Clinical Pharmacy* 17: 660–66.

Craig, W. A., et al. 1978. Hospital use of antimicrobial drugs. *Annals of Internal Medicine* 89: 793–95.

Cummings, S. R., et al. 1985. Epidemiology of osteoporosis and osteoporotic fractures. *Epidemiologic Reviews* 7: 178–208.

Darnell, J. C., et al. 1986. Medication use by ambulatory elderly: An in-home survey. *Journal of the American Geriatrics Society* 34: 1–4.

Davies, R. K. 1971. Confusional episodes and antidepressant medication. *American Journal of Psychiatry* 128: 95–99.

Davis, K., and D. Rowland. 1986. *Medicare policy: New directions for health and long-term care.* Baltimore, Md.: Johns Hopkins University Press.

Davis, M. S. 1968. Physiologic, psychological, and demographic factors in patient compliance with doctors' orders. *Medical Care* 6: 115–22.

Deberry, P., L. P. Jefferies, and M. R. Light. 1974. Teaching cardiac patients to manage medications. *American Journal of Nursing* 75: 2191–93.

DeSimone, E. M., C. F. Peterson, B. C. Carlstedt. 1977. Pharmacist-patient interaction and patient expectations. *American Journal of Pharmaceutical Education* 416: 167–71.

Dickey, F. F., M. E. Mattar, and G. M. Chudzek. 1975. Pharmacist counseling increases drug regimen compliance. *Hospitals* 49: 85–88.

Dirckx, J. H. 1979. Labels for prescribed drugs. Letter. *Journal of the American Medical Association* 242: 413–14.

Donabedian, A., and L. S. Rosenfeld. 1964. Follow-up study of chronically ill patients discharged from hospital. *Journal of Chronic Disorders* 17: 847–62.

Dunnell, K., and A. Cartwright. 1972. *Medicine takers, prescribers, and hoarders*. London: Routledge and Kegan Paul.

Ebersole, P., and P. Hess. 1981. *Toward healthy aging: Human needs and nursing response*. St. Louis, Mo.: C. V. Mosby.

The Economist. 1985. An anti-depressant for America's drug industry. Jan. 12, 1985, pp. 70–71.

Edlavitch, S. A., M. Feinleib, and C. Anello. 1985. A potential use of the national death index for postmarketing drug surveillance. *Journal of the American Medical Association* 253: 1292–95.

Eichna, L. 1983. A medical-school curriculum for the 1980s. *New England Journal of Medicine* 308: 18–21.

Engel, G. 1977. The need for a new medical model: A challenge for biomedicine. *Science* 196: 129–36.

Epstein, M. 1979. Effects of aging on the kidney. *Federation Proceedings* 38: 168–72.

Eraker, S. A., J. P. Kirscht, and M. H. Becker. 1984. Understanding and improving patient compliance. *Annals of Internal Medicine* 100: 258–68.

Estes, C. L. 1979. *The aging enterprise*. San Francisco: Jossey-Bass.

Estes, C. L., and P. C. Weiler. Health professions education for the care of the elderly: The role of the academic health center. In *Aging and the academic health center*, ed. J. Hogness. New York: Wiley. In press.

Estes, C. L., L. E. Gerard, and A. Clarke. 1984. Women and the economics of aging. In *Readings in the political economy of aging*, eds. M. Minkler and C. L. Estes. Farmingdale, N.Y.: Baywood.

Eve, S. B., and H. J. Friedsam. 1982. Use of tranquilizers and sleeping pills among older Texans. In *Drugs, alcohol, and aging*, eds. D. M. Petersen and F. J. Whittington, pp. 55–63. Dubuque, Ia.: Kendall/Hunt.

Everitt, D. E., and J. Avorn. 1986. Drug prescribing for the elderly. *Archives of Internal Medicine* 46: 2393–96.

Faich, G. A. 1986. Special report. Adverse-drug-reaction monitoring. *New England Journal of Medicine* 314: 1589–92.

Faich, G. A., et al. 1987. Reassurance about generic drugs. *New England Journal of Medicine* 316: 1473–75.

Farley, H. T. 1982. Pharmaceutical assistance for the elderly: Experiences in four states and New York. An issue paper. Mimeo. Aug. 1982.

FDA Drug Bulletin. 1982. Rockville, Md.: Department of Health and Human Services, Apr. 1982.

Federal Register. 1972. Notice of proposed rulemaking. Legal status of approved labeling of prescription drugs: Prescribing for uses unapproved by the Food and Drug Administration. 37: 16.503.

Federal Register. 1974. Conditions of participation—Pharmaceutical services. 39: 12, 17.

Feinberg, M. 1980a. Elder-Ed. *American Pharmacy* N520: 24–25.

————. 1980b. Retired pharmacists serve the elderly. *Maryland Pharmacist* 56: 6–7.

Feller, B. A. 1983. Americans needing help to function at home. *Advance data from vital and health statistics*, No. 92. DHHS Pub. No. (PHS) 83-1250. Hyattsville, Md.: National Center for Health Statistics.

Fineberg, H. V., and L. A. Pearlman. 1982. Low-cost medical practices. *Annual Review of Public Health* 3: 225–48.

Fingerhut, L. S., and H. M. Rosenberg. 1984. Mortality among the elderly. In *Health: United States, 1981*. Washington, D.C.: U.S. Department of Health and Human Services, 1981, p. 77. Cited in Bonanno and Wetle, 1984, p. 42.

Fisher, C. R. 1980. Differences by age groups in health care spending. *Health Care Financing Review 1*, Spring 1980, pp. 65–90.

Fletcher, S., E. Pappius, and S. Harper. 1979. Measurement of medication compliance in a clinical setting. *Archives of Internal Medicine* 139: 635–38.

Francis, V., B. M. Korsch, and M. J. Morris. 1969. Gaps in doctor-patient communication: Patients' response to medical advice. *New England Journal of Medicine* 280: 535–40.

Freidson, E. 1960. Client control and medical practice. *American Journal of Sociology* 65: 374–82.

————. 1973. Prepaid group practice and the new "demanding" patient. *Milbank Memorial Fund Quarterly* 51: 473–88.

Freshnock, L. 1983. Report on the 1983 PMI marketing survey. Survey and Opinion Research, American Medical Association. Mimeo. July 27, 1983.

Friedman, S. A., et al. 1972. Functional defects in the aging kidney. *Annals of Internal Medicine* 76: 41–45.

Fries, J. F. 1980. Aging, natural death, and the compression of morbidity. *New England Journal of Medicine* 303: 130–35.

Frisk, P. A., J. W. Cooper, and N. A. Campbell. 1977. Community-hospital pharmacist detection of drug-related problems upon patient admission to small hospitals. *American Journal of Hospital Pharmacy* 34: 738–42.

Fuller, M. M., and C. A. Martin. 1980. *The older woman.* Springfield, Ill.: C. C. Thomas.

Gabriel, M., J. P. Gagnon, and C. K. Bryan. 1977. Improved patient compliance through use of a daily drug reminder chart. *American Journal of Public Health* 67: 968–69.

Gagnon, J. P., E. J. Salber, and S. B. Greene. 1978. Patterns of prescription and nonprescription drug use in a southern rural area. *Public Health Reports* 93: 433–37.

Gale, J., and B. Livesley. 1974. Attitudes towards geriatrics. *Age and Ageing* 3: 49–53.

Geweke, J., and B. A. Weisbrod. 1982. Expenditure effects of technological change: The case of a new drug. Manuscript from the Department of Economics, University of Wisconsin, Madison, 1982. Cited in *Technology and Aging in America.* Washington, D.C.: U.S. Congress, Office of Technology Assessment, OTA-BA-264, June 1985, p. 138.

Gibson, R. M. 1980. National health expenditures, 1979. *Health Care Financing Review* 2, Summer 1980, pp. 1–36.

Gibson, R. M., and D. R. Waldo. 1982. National health expenditures, 1981. *Health Care Financing Review* 4, Fall 1980, pp. 1–35.

Gibson, R. M., D. R. Waldo, and K. R. Levit. 1983. National health expenditures, 1982. *Health Care Financing Review* 5, Fall 1983, pp. 1–31.

Ginsburg, P., and M. Curtis. 1978. Choice of demand parameters for CBO NHI cost estimates. U.S. Congress, Congressional Budget Office. Mimeo.

Ginzberg, E. 1985. *The U.S. health care system: A look to the 1990s.* Totowa, N.J.: Rowman & Allanheld.

Glarmet-Lenoir, C., and L. Hérisson. 1980. *La consommation pharmaceutique en France et aux USA, 1690–1978.* Paris: CREDOC (Centre de Recherche pour l'Étude et l'Observation des Conditions de Vie).

Glazer, G. B., and R. T. Zawadski. 1982. Use of psychotropic drugs among the aged, revisited. In *Drugs, alcohol, and aging,* eds. D. M. Petersen and F. J. Whittington, pp. 85–88. Dubuque, Ia.: Kendall/Hunt.

Goldberg, T., and C. A. DeVito. 1983. The impact of state generic drug substitution laws. In *Society and medication: Conflicting signals for prescribers and patients,* eds. J. P. Morgan and D. V. Kagan, pp. 99–110. Lexington, Mass.: D. C. Heath, Lexington Books.

Goldberg, T., C. A. DeVito, and T. E. Raskin, eds. 1986. *Generic drug laws: A decade of trial—A prescription for progress.* U.S. Department of Health and Human Services, Public Health Service, National Center for Health Services Research and Health Care Technology Assessment, June 1986.

Goldberg, T., et al. 1976. Evaluation of the impact of drug substitution legislation. *Journal of the American Pharmaceutical Association* NS16: 64–70, 90.

Gonzales, E. R., et al. 1984. Drugs and the elderly: When, why, how much? *Medical World News*, Jan. 23, 1984, pp. 72–74, 79–80, 85–86, 91–94.

Goodman, L. S., and A. Gilman, eds. 1970. *Pharmacological basis of therapeutics*. 4th ed. New York: Macmillan.

Gordis, L., M. Markowitz, and A. M. Lilienfeld. 1969. Studies in the epidemiology and preventability of rheumatic fever. *Pediatrics* 43: 173–82.

Graham, H., and B. Livesley. 1983. Can readmissions to a geriatric medical unit be prevented? *Lancet* 1: 404–6.

Greenblatt, D. J., M. D. Allen, and R. I. Shader. 1977. Toxicity of high dose flurazepam in the elderly. *Clinical Pharmacology and Therapeutics* 21: 355–61.

Greenblatt, D. J., E. M. Sellers, and R. I. Shader. 1982. Drug disposition in old age. *New England Journal of Medicine* 306: 1081–88.

Guglielmo, B. J., et al. 1986. Daily drug costs in treating infection. Antibiotic Advisory Subcommittee Newsletter, University of California, San Francisco Medical Center, July 1986.

Gundert-Remy, U., C. Remy, and E. Weber. 1976. Serum digoxin levels in patients of a general practice of Germany. *European Journal of Clinical Pharmacology* 10: 97–100.

Guttmann, D. 1977. *A survey of drug taking behavior in the elderly*. U.S. Department of Health, Education, and Welfare.

Hale, W. E., R. G. Marks, and R. B. Stewart. 1979. Drug use in a geriatric population. *Journal of the American Geriatrics Society* 27: 374–77.

———. 1980. The dunedin program, a Florida geriatric screening process: Design and initial data. *Journal of the American Geriatrics Society* 27: 377–80.

Hammarlund, E. R., J. R. Ostrom, and A. J. Kethley. 1985. The effects of drug counseling and other educational strategies on drug utilization of the elderly. *Medical Care* 23: 165–70.

Hanson, A. L. 1981. An external doctor of pharmacy degree. *Möbius* 1: 35–45.

Hansten, P. D. 1986. Harmful drug-drug interactions. In *Topics in clinical pharmacology and therapeutics*, ed. R. F. Maronde, pp. 382–86. New York: Springer-Verlag.

Hare, E. H., and D. R. Willcox. 1967. Do psychiatric inpatients take their pills? *British Journal of Psychiatry* 113: 1435–39.

Harper, A., L. H. Butler, and P. W. Newacheck. 1980. Health maintenance organizations and the elderly. *Home Health Care Services Quarterly* 1: 81–97.

Harris, R., M. W. Linn, and B. S. Linn. 1981. Psychotropic drugs in the ambulatory care of elderly males. *Medical Care* 19: 930–35.

Hartshorn, E. 1976. Interactions of CNS antidepressant psychotherapeutic agents. In *Handbook of drug interactions*, 3d ed., pp. 130–35. Hamilton, Ill.: Hamilton Press, Drug Intelligence Publications.

Haug, M. R. 1979. Doctor-patient relationships and the older patient. *Journal of Gerontology* 34: 852–60.

Haug, M. R., ed. 1981. *Elderly patients and their doctors*. New York: Springer.

Haug, M. R., and B. Lavin. 1979. Public challenge of physician authority. *Medical Care* 17: 844–58.

Haynes, R. B. 1976. A critical review of the "determinants" of patient compliance with therapeutic regimens. In *Compliance with therapeutic regimens*, eds. D. L. Sackett and R. B. Haynes, pp. 26–50. Baltimore, Md.: Johns Hopkins University Press.

Haynes, R. B., D. L. Sackett, and D. W. Taylor. 1980. How to detect and manage low patient compliance in chronic illness. *Geriatrics* 355: 91–97.

Haynes, R. B., et al. 1982. Process versus outcome in hypertension: A positive result. *Circulation* 65: 28–33.

Health and Public Policy Committee, American College of Physicians. 1983. Drug therapy for severe, chronic pain in terminal illness. *Annals of Internal Medicine* 99: 870–73.

Hearing before Subcommittee on Health and the Environment. 1985. Committee on Energy and Commerce, House of Representatives, 99th Congress, July 15, 1985.

Heath, C. 1980. On prescription writing in social interaction. In *Prescribing practice and drug usage*, ed. R. Mapes, pp. 58–69. London: Croom Helm.

Hemminki, E. 1975. Review of literature on the factors affecting drug prescribing. *Social Science and Medicine* 9: 111–15.

Hemminki, E., and J. Heikkila. 1975. Elderly people's compliance with prescriptions and quality of medication. *Scandinavian Journal of Social Medicine* 3: 87–92.

Herfindal, E. T., L. R. Bernstein, and D. T. Kishi. 1983. Effect of clinical pharmacy services in prescribing on an orthopedic unit. *American Journal of Hospital Pharmacy* 40: 1945–51.

Herxheimer, A. 1977. L'Automédication. In *Thérapeutique médicale*, eds. P. Fèbre, et al. Paris: Flammarion.

Hill, I. T. 1987. *Broadening Medicaid coverage of pregnant women and children: State policy responses*. Washington, D.C.: State Medicaid Information Center, National Governors Association.

Hodgson, T. A., and A. N. Kopstein. 1984. Health expenditures for major diseases in 1980. *Health Care Financing Review* 5, Summer 1984, pp. 1–12.

Hoffman, R. P. 1978. Anti-infective utilization review in a community hospital. *Hospital Pharmacy* 13: 461–80.

Holahan, J. F., and J. W. Cohen. 1986. *Medicaid: The trade-off between cost containment and access to care*. Washington, D.C.: Urban Institute Press.

Hulka, B. S., et al. 1975. Medication use and misuse: Physician-patient discrepancies. *Journal of Chronic Diseases* 28: 7–21.

Hulka, B. S., et al. 1976. Communication, compliance, and concordance between physicians and patients with prescribed medications. *American Journal of Public Health* 66: 847–53.

Hulse, R. K., et al. 1976. Computerized medication monitoring system. *American Journal of Hospital Pharmacy* 33: 1061–64.

Hurwitz, N. 1969. Predisposing factors to adverse drug reactions. *British Medical Journal* 1: 536–39.

Hussar, D. A. 1975. Patient noncompliance. *Journal of the American Pharmaceutical Association* 15: 183–90, 201.

Hutt, P. B. 1980. The legal requirement that drugs be proved safe and effective before their use. In *Controversies in therapeutics*, ed. L. Lasagna, pp. 495–506. Philadelphia: W. B. Saunders.

Iglehart, J. K. 1985. Medicare turns to HMOs. Health Policy Report, *New England Journal of Medicine* 312: 132–36.

Institute of Medicine. 1978. *Aging and medical education.* Washington, D.C.: National Academy of Sciences.

———. 1979. *Sleeping pills, insomnia, and medical practice.* Washington, D.C.: National Academy of Sciences.

Institute on Aging, Work, and Health. 1985. *Post-retirement medical benefit: Survey report.* Washington, D.C.: Washington Business Group on Health, June 1985.

Interstudy. 1986. *Improving health and long-term care for the elderly.* Excelsior, Minn.: 1–78.

Inui, T. S., J. W. Yourtee, and J. W. Williamson. 1976. Improved outcomes in hypertension after physician tutorials: A controlled trial. *Annals of Internal Medicine* 84: 646–51.

Irvine, R. D., et al. 1974. The effect of age on the hydroxylation of amylobarbitone sodium in man. *British Journal of Clinical Pharmacology* 1: 41–43.

Irwin, D. S., W. D. Weitzell, and D. W. Morgan. 1971. Phenothiazine intake and staff attitudes. *American Journal of Psychiatry* 127: 1631–35.

Javert, C., and C. Macri. 1941. Prothrombin concentration and mineral oil. *American Journal of Obstetrics and Gynecology*, June 1941, pp. 409–14.

Jefferys, M., J. H. F. Brotherston, and A. Cartwright. 1960. Consumption of medicines on a working-class housing estate. *British Journal of Preventive and Social Medicine* 14: 64–76.

Jick, H. 1974. Drugs—remarkably non-toxic. *New England Journal of Medicine* 291: 824–28.

———. Adverse drug reactions. 1986. In *Topics in clinical pharmacology and therapeutics*, ed. R. F. Maronde, pp. 397–404. New York: Springer-Verlag.

Jick, H., et al. 1968. Efficacy and toxicity of heparin in relation to age and sex. *New England Journal of Medicine* 279: 284–86.

Jick, H., et al. 1970. Comprehensive drug surveillance. *Journal of the American Medical Association* 213: 1455–60.

Johnson, R. E., and D. J. Azevedo. 1979. Examining the annual drug utilization of a cohort of low-income health plan members. *Medical Care* 17: 578–91.

Joint Commission on Prescription Drug Use. 1980. *Final report and appendices I through XI*. Rockville, Md.: Joint Commission on Prescription Drug Use, Jan. 23, 1980.

Joubert, P., and L. Lasagna. 1975. Patient package inserts: Nature, notions, and needs. *Clinical Pharmacology and Therapeutics* 18: 507.

Kalimo, E. 1969. *Determinants of medical care utilization: Correlational multivariate analyses of illness behavior and the factors affecting it among the adult population of Finland prior to the national sickness insurance scheme*. Helsinki: Research Institute for Social Security.

Kane, R. L., J. G. Ouslander, and I. B. Abrass, eds. 1984. *Essentials of clinical geriatrics*. New York: McGraw-Hill.

Kane, R. L., et al. 1980a. The future need for geriatric manpower in the United States. *New England Journal of Medicine* 302: 1327–32.

———. 1980b. *Geriatrics in the United States: Manpower projections and training considerations*. Santa Monica, Calif.: Rand Corporation.

———. 1981. *Geriatrics in the United States*. Lexington, Mass.: D. C. Heath, Lexington Books.

Kanouse, D. E., et al. 1981. *Informing patients about drugs: Summary report on alternative designs for prescription drug leaflets*. Santa Monica, Calif.: Rand Corporation.

Karasu, T. B., et al. 1979. Age factors in the patient-therapist relationship. *Journal of Nervous and Mental Disorders* 167: 100–104.

Karsh, F. E. 1980. Is drug toxicity a problem of great magnitude? Probably not. In *Controversies in therapeutics*, ed. L. Lasagna, pp. 51–57. Philadelphia: W. B. Saunders.

Kasper, J. A. 1982. Prescribed medicines: Use, expenditures, and sources of payment. In *Data Preview 9: National Health Care Expenditure Study*, DHHS Pub. No. (PHS) 82-3320, U.S. Department of Health and Human Services, Apr. 1, 1982.

Kasper, J. A., et al. 1980. Expenditures for personal health services: Findings from the 1977 national medical care expenditure survey. Paper presented to 108th Annual American Public Health Association meeting in Detroit, Mich., Oct. 21, 1980.

Keeler, E. B., et al. 1982. Effect of patient age in duration of medical encounters with physicians. *Medical Care* 20: 1101–8.

Kelly, J. F. 1986. Clinical pharmacology of chemotherapeutic agents in old age. In *Cancer and the elderly, frontiers of radiation therapy and oncology*, eds. J. M. Vaeth and J. Meyer, Vol. 20, pp. 101–11. Basel: S. Karger.

Keys, P. W., J. C. South, and M. G. Duffy. 1975. Quality of care evaluation applied to assessment of clinical pharmacy services. *American Journal of Hospital Pharmacy* 32: 897–902.

Klein, L. E., P. S. German, and D. M. Levine. 1981. Adverse drug reactions among the elderly: A reassessment. *Journal of the American Geriatrics Society* 29: 525–30.

Klein, L. E., et al. 1982. Aging and its relationship to health knowledge and medication compliance. *Gerontologist* 22: 384–87.

Knapp, D. A. 1974. *Consumers and medicine.* Springfield, Va.: National Technical Information Service.

———. 1978. Can pharmacists influence drug prescribing? *American Journal of Hospital Pharmacy* 35: 593.

Knapp, D. A., and D. E. Knapp. 1972. Decision-making and self-medication: Preliminary findings. *American Journal of Hospital Pharmacy* 29: 1004–12.

———. 1980. The elderly and non-prescribed medications. *Contemporary Pharmacy Practice* 3: 85–89.

Koch, H. 1982. Drug utilization in office practice by age and sex of the patient: National Ambulatory Medical Care Survey, 1980. In *Advance Data from Vital and Health Statistics*, No. 81. DHHS Pub. No. (PHS) 82-1250. Hyattsville, Md.: National Center for Health Statistics.

———. 1983. Utilization of psychotropic drugs in office-based ambulatory care: National Ambulatory Medical Care Survey, 1980 and 1981. In *Advance Data from Vital and Health Statistics*, No. 90. DHHS Pub. No. (PHS) 83-1250. Hyattsville, Md.: National Center for Health Statistics.

Koch, H., and M. C. Smith. 1985. Office-based ambulatory care for patients 75 years old and over: National Ambulatory Medical Care Survey, 1980 and 1981. In *Advance Data from Vital and Health Statistics*, No. 110. DHHS Pub. No. (PHS) 85-1250. Hyattsville, Md.: National Center for Health Statistics.

Koos, E. L. 1954. *The health of Regionville.* New York: Hafner.

Korsch, B., and V. Negrete. 1972. Doctor-patient communication. *Scientific American* 227: 66–74.

Kovar, M. G. 1977. *Health United States, 1976–1977.* DHEW Pub. No. (HRA) 77-1232, U.S. Department of Health, Education, and Welfare. Washington, D.C.: Government Printing Office.

———. 1983. The United States—Elderly people and their medical care. Background Paper for Commonwealth Fund Forum on Improving the Health of the Homebound Elderly, London, May 1983.

Kroczynksi, R. P. 1984. Drug purchasing: An evolutionary blueprint. *Business and Health* 1: 32–34.

Krondl, A. 1970. Present understanding of the interaction of drugs and food during absorption. *Canadian Medical Association Journal* 10: 360–64.

Kunin, C. M., T. Tupasi, and W. A. Craig. 1973. Use of antibiotics: A brief exposition of the problem and some tentative solutions. *Annals of Internal Medicine* 19: 555–60.

Kushner, D., and R. Feierman. 1985. Average Rx price tops $10, chains again outpace indeps in per-store performance. *American Druggist*, May 1985, pp. 17–18, 23, 26.

Lamy, P. P. 1979. OTC drugs and the elderly. *Current Prescribing* 11: 42–52.

———. 1980. *Prescribing for the elderly*. Littleton, Mass.: PSG Publishing.

———. 1982. Over-the-counter medication: The drug interactions we overlook. *Journal of the American Geriatrics Society* Supplement 30: S69–S75.

———. 1984. Patterns of prescribing and drug use. In *The aging process: Therapeutic implications*, eds. R. N. Butler and A. J. Bearn, pp. 53–95. New York: Raven.

———. 1986. The elderly and drug interactions. *Journal of the American Geriatrics Society* 34: 586–92.

Lamy, P. P., and R. S. Beardsley. 1982. The older adult and the pharmacist educator. *American Pharmacy* NS22: 40–42.

Lamy, P. P., and M. Feinberg. 1982. Elder-Health: Partners in care. *Maryland Pharmacist* 58: 4–22.

Lasagna, L. 1974. Bureaucratic controls will shift both industry and intelligent medical practice. In *Controversies in internal medicine II*, eds. F. J. Ingelfinger, et al., pp. 74–80. Philadelphia: W. B. Saunders.

Latiolais, C., and C. Berry. 1969. Misuse of prescription medication by outpatients. *Drug Intelligence and Clinical Pharmacy* 3: 270–77.

LaVange, L., and H. Silverman. 1987. Outpatient prescription drug utilization and expenditure patterns of noninstitutionalized aged Medicare beneficiaries. *National Medical Care Utilization and Expenditure Survey*, Series B, Descriptive Report No. 12. DHHS Pub. No. 85-20212. Office of Research and Demonstrations, Health Care Financing Administration. Washington, D.C.: Government Printing Office.

Leadership Council of Aging Organizations. 1983. *The administration's 1984 budget: A critical view from an aging perspective*. Washington, D.C.: Leadership Council of Aging Organizations, Mar. 15, 1983.

Learoyd, B. M. 1972. Psychotropic drugs and the elderly patient. *Medical Journal of Australia* 22: 1131–33.

Lech, S. V., G. D. Freidman, and H. K. Ury. 1975. Characteristics of heavy users of outpatient prescription drugs. *Clinical Toxicology* 8: 599–610.

Lee, A. J., et al. 1983. Evaluation of the maximum allowable cost program. *Health Care Financing Review* 4, Spring 1983, pp. 71–82.

Lee, P. R. 1979. Prescription drug use and patient education—The critical role of the pharmacist. *American Journal of Pharmaceutical Education* 43: 354–57.

———. 1980a. America is an overmedicated society. In *Controversies in therapeutics*, ed. L. Lasagna. Philadelphia: W. B. Saunders.

————. 1980b. Medication and prescribing. In *Primary care*, ed. J. Fry, pp. 230–51. London: Heinemann.

————. 1981a. *Drugs, drug information, and drug information systems: The need for a national policy*. In Proceedings of the Hawaii International Conference on System Science, Vol. II, pp. 230–51. Honolulu: University of Hawaii Press.

————. 1981b. Pills, profits, and politics. Speech given at the School of Public Health, University of California, Los Angeles, Jan. 29, 1981.

————. 1986. Cost containment: Economics and policy issues. In *Cancer and the elderly: Frontiers of radiation therapy and oncology*, eds. J. M. Vaeth and J. Meyers, Vol. 20, pp. 58–68. Basel: S. Karger.

Lee, P. R., and C. L. Estes. 1979. Eighty federal programs for the elderly. In *The aging enterprise*, ed. C. L. Estes. San Francisco: Jossey-Bass.

Lee, P. R., and H. L. Lipton. 1983. *Drugs and the elderly*. A background paper. Prepared for the Administration on Aging, U.S. Department of Health and Human Services, July 1983.

————. 1986. The role of drugs and the U.S. pharmaceutical industry in health care. In *Generic drug laws: A decade of trial—A prescription for progress*, eds. T. Goldberg, C. A. DeVito, and T. E. Raskin. U.S. Department of Health and Human Services, Public Health Service, National Center for Health Services Research and Health Care Technology Assessment, June 1986.

Leibowitz, A., W. J. Manning, and J. P. Newhouse. 1985. The demand for prescription drugs as a function of cost-sharing. *Social Science and Medicine* 21: 1063–69.

Lennox, K. 1979. *Prescription drugs*, Vol. 2. Washington, D.C.: Urban Institute.

Levin, L. S., and E. L. Idler. 1981. *The hidden health care system: Mediating structures and medicine*. Cambridge, Mass.: Ballinger.

Levit, K. R., et al. 1985. National health expenditures, 1984. *Health Care Financing Review* 7, Fall 1985, pp. 1–35.

Lewis, C. E., and M. Michnich. 1977. Contracts as a means of improving patient compliance. In *Medication compliance: A behavioral management approach*, ed. I. Barofsky, pp. 69–75. Thorofare, N.J.: Charles B. Slack.

Lexchin, J. 1986. Determinants of physician prescribing patterns and behavior. Cited in *Generic drug laws: A decade of trial—A prescription for progress*, eds. T. Goldberg, C. A. DeVito, and T. E. Raskin, pp. 71–98. U.S. Department of Health and Human Services, Public Health Service, National Center for Health Services Research and Health Care Technology Assessment, June 1986.

Lindeman, R. D., J. Tobin, and N. W. Shock. 1985. Longitudinal studies on the rate of decline in renal function with age. *Journal of the American Geriatrics Society* 33: 278–85.

Link, G., and K. Feiden. 1978. How 12 San Francisco RPh's curb drug misuse by the elderly. *American Druggist*, Dec. 1978, pp. 28–29, 33.

Linkewich, J. A., R. B. Catalano, and H. L. Hack. 1974. The effect of packaging and instruction on outpatient compliance with medication regimens. *Drug Intelligence and Clinical Pharmacy* 8: 10–15.

Linn, L. S. 1971. Physician characteristics and attitudes toward legitimate use of psychotherapeutic drugs. *Journal of Health and Social Behavior* 12: 132–40.

Lipton, H. 1982. The graying of America: Implications for the pharmacist. *American Journal of Hospital Pharmacy* 39: 131–35.

———. 1987. Prescription drugs and the elderly—The high cost of growing old. Statement before the U.S. Senate Special Committee on Aging. Washington, D.C., July 20, 1987.

Lipton, H., and B. L. Svarstad. 1974. Parental expectations of a multidisciplinary clinic for children with developmental disabilities. *Journal of Health and Social Behavior* 15: 157–66.

Little, Arthur D., Inc. 1984a. Beta-blocker reduction of mortality and reinfarction rate in survivors of myocardial infarction: A cost-benefit study. *Cost-effectiveness of pharmaceuticals* Report Series, Report 7. Pharmaceutical Manufacturers Association, Apr. 1984.

———. 1984b. Use of a beta-blocker in the treatment of glaucoma: A cost-benefit study. *Cost-effectiveness of pharmaceuticals* Report Series, Report 8. Pharmaceutical Manufacturers Association, Apr. 1984.

———. 1984c. Use of beta-blockers in the treatment of angina: A cost-benefit study. *Cost-effectiveness of pharmaceuticals* Report Series, Report 9. Pharmaceutical Manufacturers Association, Apr. 1984.

Lofholm, P. 1978. Self-medication by the elderly. In *Drugs and the elderly*, ed. R. C. Kayne, pp. 8–28. Los Angeles, Calif.: University of Southern California Press.

Loomis, M. T., and T. F. Williams. 1983. Evaluation of care provided to terminally ill patients. *Gerontologist* 23: 493–99.

Lowenstine, F. W. 1982. Nutritional status of the elderly in the United States of America. *Journal of the American College of Nutrition* 1: 165–77.

Luft, H. 1981. *Health maintenance organizations: Dimensions of performance.* New York: Wiley.

Luger, S. 1984. An alternative reimbursement system to encourage optimum pharmacy services. *American Health Care Association Journal* 10: 11–16.

Lundin, D. V. 1978. Medication taking behavior of the elderly: A pilot study. *Drug Intelligence and Clinical Pharmacy* 12: 518–22.

Lundin, D. V., et al. 1980. Education of independent elderly in the responsible use of prescription medications. *Drug Intelligence and Clinical Pharmacy* 14: 335–42.

McCall, N., and S. Rice. 1981. *Evaluation of the Colorado clinical psychology/ expanded mental health benefits experiment.* Executive Summary. Baltimore, Md.: Office of Research, Demonstrations, and Statistics, Health Care Financing Administration. May 1981.

MacDonald, E. T., J. B. MacDonald, and M. Phoenix. 1977. Improving drug compliance after hospital discharge. *British Medical Journal* 2: 618–21.

MacDonald, J. 1984. The role of drugs in falls in the elderly. In *Biological and behavioral aspects of falls in the elderly.* Proceedings of a conference sponsored by the National Institute on Aging, Sept. 17–18, 1984.

MacDonald, J., and E. MacDonald. 1977. Nocturnal femoral fractures and continuing widespread use of barbiturate hypnotics. *British Medical Journal* 2: 483–85.

McCrae, R. R., and P. T. Costa. 1984. *Emerging lives, enduring dispositions: Personality in adulthood.* Boston: Little, Brown.

McGhan, W. F., et al. 1983. A comparison of pharmacists and physicians on the quality of prescribing for ambulatory hypertensive patients. *Medical Care* 21: 435–53.

McKenney, J., and W. L. Harrison. 1976. Drug-related hospital admissions. *American Journal of Hospital Pharmacy* 33: 792–95.

McKenney, J. M., et al. 1973. The effect of clinical pharmacy services on patients with essential hypertension. *Circulation* 48: 1104–11.

McKenney, J. M., et al. 1978. Effect of pharmacist drug monitoring and patient education on hypertensive patients. *Contemporary Pharmacy Practice* 1: 50–56.

McNeely, R. L., ed. 1983. *Aging in minority groups.* Beverly Hills, Calif.: Sage.

Madden, E. E. 1973. Evaluation of outpatient pharmacy counseling. *Journal of the American Pharmaceutical Association* NS13: 437–43.

Maddox, G. L. 1979. Drugs, physicians, and patients. In *Drugs and the elderly,* eds. D. M. Petersen, F. J. Whittington, and B. P. Payne, pp. 5–27. Springfield, Ill.: Charles C. Thomas.

Makarushka, J. L., and R. W. McDonald. 1979. Informed consent, research, and geriatric patients: The responsibility of institutional review committees. *Gerontologist* 19: 61–66.

Maki, D. G., and A. A. Schuna. 1978. A study of antimicrobial misuse in a university hospital. *American Journal of Medical Science* 275: 271–82.

Malahay, B. 1966. The effect of instruction and labeling on the number of medication errors made by patients at home. *American Journal of Hospital Pharmacy* 23: 283–92.

Manning, P., et al. 1980. Determining educational needs in the physician's office. *Journal of the American Medical Association* 244: 1112–15.

Manton, K. C. 1982. Changing concepts of morbidity and mortality in the elderly population. *Milbank Memorial Fund Quarterly/Health and Society*, Spring 1982, pp. 183–245.

Marks, R. M., and E. J. Sachar. 1973. Undertreatments of medical inpatients with narcotic analgesics. *Annals of Internal Medicine* 78: 173–81.

Maronde, R. F. 1971. Drug utilization review with on-line computer capacity. Los Angeles County General Hospital and University of Southern California School of Medicine, DHEW Publication No. (SSA) 73-11853, Staff Paper 13.

———. 1977. Drug utilization review. In *Perspectives on medicines in society*, eds. A. I. Wertheimer and P. J. Bush, pp. 169–91. Hamilton, Ill.: Drug Intelligence Publications.

Marttila, J. K., et al. 1977. Potential untoward effects of long-term use of flurazepam in geriatric patients. *Journal of the American Pharmaceutical Association* NS17: 692–95.

Mattar, M. E., J. Markello, and S. J. Jaffe. 1975. Pharmaceutic factors affecting pediatric compliance. *Pediatrics* 55: 101–8.

May, F. E., R. B. Stewart, and L. E. Cluff. 1974. Drug use in the hospital: Evaluation of determinants. *Clinical Pharmacology and Therapeutics* 16: 834–45.

May, F. E., et al. 1982. Prescribed and nonprescribed drug use in an ambulatory elderly population. *Southern Medical Journal* 75: 522–28.

Mazulla, J. M., L. Lasagna, and P. F. Griner. 1974. Variations in interpretation of prescription instructions. *Journal of the American Medical Association* 227: 929–31.

Mellinger, G. D., and M. B. Balter. 1981. Prevalence and patterns of use of psychotherapeutic drugs: Results from a 1979 national survey of American adults. In *Proceedings of the International Seminar on Epidemiological Impact of Psychotropic Drugs*, eds. G. Tognoni, C. Bellantuono, and M. Lader, pp. 117–35. Milan, Amsterdam: Elsevier/North-Holland Biomedical Press.

Mellinger, G. D., M. Balter, and D. Manheimer. 1971. Patterns of psychotherapeutic drug use among adults in San Francisco. *Archives of General Psychiatry* 25: 385–94.

Mellinger, G. D., M. B. Balter, and E. H. Uhlenhuth. 1984. Prevalence and correlates of the long-term regular use of anxiolytics. *Journal of the American Medical Association* 251: 375–79.

Melmon, K. 1974. Preventable drug reactions: Causes and cures. *New England Journal of Medicine* 284: 1361–68.

Melmon, K. L., and T. F. Blaschke. 1983. The undereducated physician's therapeutic decisions. *New England Journal of Medicine* 308: 1473–74.

Miles, L. E., and W. C. Dement. 1980. Sleep and aging. *Sleep* 3: 119–220.

Miller, D. B., et al. 1976. Physicians' attitudes towards the ill, aged, and nursing homes. *Journal of the American Geriatrics Society* 24: 498–505.

Miller, M. D. 1946. *Elements of graduation.* Actuarial Monographs No. 1. Chicago: Actuarial Society of America, American Institute of Actuaries.

Miller, R. R. 1973. Drug surveillance utilizing epidemiologic methods. A report from the Boston Collaborative Drug Surveillance Program. *American Journal of Hospital Pharmacy* 30: 584–92.

Miller, R. W. 1983. Doctors, patients don't communicate. *FDA Consumer* 17, July/Aug. 1983, pp. 6–7.

Miller, S. J. 1984. A survey of nationwide health maintenance organizations. Department of Pharmacy Practice and Administrative Science, School of Pharmacy, University of Maryland. Dec. 1984. Mimeo.

Milleren, J. W. 1977. Some contingencies affecting the utilization of tranquilizers in long-term care of the elderly. *Journal of Health and Social Behavior* 18: 206–11.

Millstein, L. G. 1984. Issues in geriatric labeling revisions. Paper presented at the Drug Information Association Meeting, Washington, D.C., Feb. 27, 1984.

Moore, S. R. 1983. *Final report of Working Group on Drug Use and Misuse in the Elderly.* U.S. Department of Health and Human Services, Public Health Service, June 3, 1983. Mimeo.

Moore, S. R., M. Kalu, and R. Yavaprabbas. 1983. Receipt of prescription drug information by the elderly. *Drug Intelligence and Clinical Pharmacy* 17: 920–23.

Morris, L. A., and J. Halperin. 1979. Effects of written drug information on patient knowledge and compliance: A literature review. *American Journal of Public Health* 69: 47–52.

Morris, L. A., and N. J. Olins. 1984. Utility of drug leaflets for elderly consumers. *American Journal of Public Health* 74: 157–58.

Morris, L. A., et al. 1977. A survey of the effects of oral contraceptive patient information. *Journal of the American Medical Association* 238: 2504–8.

Moser, R. H. 1964. *Diseases of medical progress.* Springfield, Ill.: Charles Thomas.

———. 1974. The continuing search: FDA drug information survey. *Journal of the American Medical Association* 229: 1336–38.

Moulding, T. S. 1979. The unrealized potential of the medication monitor. *Clinical Pharmacology and Therapeutics* 25: 131–36.

Mueller, C. 1972. The overmedicated society: Forces in the marketplace for medical care. *Science* 176: 488.

Muller, C. 1968. Outpatient drug prescribing related to clinic utilization in four New York City hospitals. *Health Services Research* 3: 142–54.

Murray, R. M. 1973. Patterns of analgesic use and abuse in medical patients. *Practitioner* 211: 639–44.

Musher, D. M., E. J. Young, and R. J. Hamill. 1986. The ethics of pharmaceutical promotion. Letter to the editor. *New England Journal of Medicine* 315: 590.

The Nation. Drug topics, Jan. 3, 1980, p. 1.

National Academy of Engineering, Committee on Technology and International Economic and Trade Issues, Pharmaceutical Panel. 1982. *The competitive status of the U.S. pharmaceutical industry: A study of the determining international industrial competitive advantage* (draft). Washington, D.C.: National Academy of Engineering.

National Analysts, Inc. 1972. *A study of health practices and opinions.* Philadelphia: National Analysts.

National Center for Health Statistics. 1985. Current estimates from the National Health Interview Survey: United States, 1982. *Vital and Health Statistics* Series 10, No. 150, DHHS Pub. No. (PHS) 85-1578. Washington, D.C.: Government Printing Office, Sept. 1985.

National Center for Health Statistics, and B. Bloom. 1982. Current estimates from the National Health Interview Survey: United States, 1981. *Vital and Health Statistics* Series 10, No. 141, DHHS Pub. No. (PHS) 83-1569. Washington, D.C.: Government Printing Office.

National Center for Health Statistics, and S. S. Jack. 1981. Current estimates from the National Health Interview Survey: United States, 1979. *Vital and Health Statistics* Series 10, No. 136, DHHS Pub. No. (PHS) 81-1564. Washington, D.C.: Government Printing Office.

National Center for Health Statistics, and P. W. Ries. 1983. Americans assess their health: 1978. *Vital and Health Statistics* Series 10, No. 142, DHHS Pub. No. (PHS) 83-1570. Washington, D.C.: Government Printing Office.

National Institute on Aging, National Institute of Health, U.S. Public Health Service, Department of Health and Human Services. 1984. *Report on education and training in geriatrics and gerontology.* Washington, D.C.: Government Printing Office.

Needleman, P., and E. M. Johnson. 1981. Vasodilators. In *The pharmacologic basis of therapeutics,* eds. A. G. Gilman, L. S. Goodman, and A. Gilman, pp. 830–31. New York: Macmillan.

Neeley, E., and M. L. Patrick. 1968. Problems of aged persons taking medications at home. *Nursing Research* 17: 52–55.

Nelson, E. L., et al. 1978. Impact of patient perceptions on compliance with treatment for hypertension. *Medical Care* 16: 893–906.

New Jersey Department of Human Services. 1985. *Pharmaceutical Assistance to the Aged and Disabled (PAAD): Fiscal year 1984 annual report.*

———. 1987. *Pharmaceutical Assistance to the Aged and Disabled (PAAD): Fiscal year 1986 annual report.*

Nightingale, S. L. 1981. Drug regulation and policy formulation. *Health and Society* 59: 412–44.

Novitch, M. 1983. Testimony delivered to a joint hearing before the Special Committee on Aging, U.S. Senate, and the Subcommittee on Health and

Long-Term Care, Select Committee on Aging, U.S. House of Representatives, June 28, 1983.

Office of National Cost Estimates, Office of the Actuary, Health Care Financing Administration. 1987. National health expenditures 1986–2000. *Health Care Financing Review* 8 (Summer): 1–36.

O'Malley, K., et al. 1971. Effect of age and sex on human drug metabolism. *British Medical Journal* 3: 607–9.

Ostrom, J. R., et al. 1985. Medication usage in an elderly population. *Medical Care* 23: 157–64.

Ouslander, J. G. 1981. Drug therapy in the elderly. *Annals of Internal Medicine* 95: 711–22.

Parkin, D., et al. 1976. Deviation from prescribed drug treatment after discharge from hospital. *British Medical Journal* 2: 686–88.

Parry, H., et al. 1973. National patterns of psychotherapeutic drug use. *Archives of General Psychiatry* 28: 769–83.

Parsons, T. 1951. *The social system*. Glencoe, Ill.: Free Press.

Pellegrino, E. D. 1976. Prescribing and drug ingestion: Symbols and substance. Paper delivered at the annual meeting, American Association for the Advancement of Science, Boston, Mass., Feb. 18–24, 1976.

Pennsylvania Blue Shield. 1985. Background paper, *The medication passport and drug education program for senior citizens*, June 1985.

Pennsylvania Department of Aging, PACE (Pharmaceutical Assistance Contract for the Elderly). 1985. *Fourth quarterly report to the Pennsylvania General Assembly*.

Petersen, D. M., F. J. Whittington, and B. P. Payne, eds. 1979. *Drugs and the elderly: Social and pharmacological issues*. Springfield, Ill.: Charles C. Thomas.

Pfeiffer, E. 1979. Role of the pharmacist in providing health services to the aged. *Pharmacy Management* 151: 85–87.

Pharmaceutical Manufacturers Association. 1984. *Cost-effectiveness of pharmaceuticals: A summary report*. Washington, D.C.: Apr. 1984.

Pharmacy Task Force, Medical Care Section, American Public Health Association. 1979. Pharmacy services under national health insurance: Justification and guiding principles. Statement prepared for annual meeting, New York, N.Y., Nov. 5, 1979.

Pharmacy Times. 1980. The top 200 drugs. 46: 31.

———. 1986. Top 200 drugs of 1985: A 1.4% increase in refills nudges 1985 Rxs 1.1% ahead of 1984 volume. 52: 25–33.

Pierpaoli, P., J. Coarse, and R. Tilton. 1976. Antibiotic use control—An institutional model. *Drug Intelligence and Clinical Pharmacy* 10: 258–67.

Plant, J. 1977. Educating the elderly in safe medication use. *Hospitals* 51: 97–102.

Podell, R., D. Kent, and K. Keller. 1976. Patient psychological defenses and physician response in the long-term treatment of hypertension. *Journal of Family Practice* 3: 145–49.

Porter, A. M. W. 1969. Drug defaulting in a general practice. *British Medical Journal* 1: 218–22.

Porter, J., and H. Jick. 1977. Drug related deaths among medical patients. *Journal of the American Medical Association* 231: 879–81.

Pratt, L. 1973. The significance of the family in medication. *Journal of Comparative Family Studies* 4: 13–32.

Prentice, R. 1979. Patterns of psychoactive drug use among the elderly. In *The aging process and psychoactive drug use*. Rockville, Md.: U.S. Department of Health, Education, and Welfare, Public Health Service, Alcohol, Drug Abuse, and Mental Health Administration, Services Research Branch, Division of Resource Development.

Quah, S. R. 1977. Self-medication: A neglected dimension of health behavior. *Sociological Symposium* 19: 28–36.

Quill, T. E. 1983. Partnerships in patient care: A contractual approach. *Annals of Internal Medicine* 98: 228–34.

Rabin, D. L. 1977. Prescribed and nonprescribed medicine use. In *Perspectives on medicines in society*, eds. A. Wertheimer and P. Bush, pp. 58–87. Hamilton, Ill.: Drug Intelligence Publications.

Rabin, D., ed. 1972. International comparisons of medical care. Preliminary report of the World Health Organization/International Collaborative Study of Medical Care Utilization. *Milbank Memorial Fund Quarterly* 50: Part 2.

Rabin, D. L., and P. J. Bush. 1974. The use of medicines: Historical trends and international comparison. *International Journal of Health Services* 4: 61–87.

———. 1975. Who's using medicines? *Journal of Community Health* 1: 106.

———. 1976. Who's using prescribed medicines? *Drugs in Health Care* 3: 89–100.

Raskind, M. A., et al. 1976. Helping the elderly psychiatric patient in crisis. *Geriatrics* 31: 51–56.

Ratzan, R. M. 1980. "Being old makes you different": The ethics of research with elderly subjects. *Hastings Center Report* 10, Oct. 1980, pp. 32–42.

Ray, W. A., C. F. Federspiel, and W. Schaffner. 1980. A study of antipsychotic drug use in nursing homes: Epidemiologic evidence suggesting misuse. *American Journal of Public Health* 70: 485–91.

Ray, W. A., et al. 1987. Psychotropic drug use and the risk of hip fracture. *New England Journal of Medicine* 316: 363–69.

Reber, A. *Nutrition and aging*. 1979. Denton: North Texas State University, Center for Studies in Aging.

Reich, W. T. 1978. Ethical issues related to research involving elderly subjects. *Gerontologist* 18: 326–37.

Reidenberg, M. M., et al. 1978. Relationship between diazepam dose, plasma level, age, and central nervous system depression. *Clinical Pharmacology and Therapeutics* 23: 371–74.

Reilly, M. J. 1970. Folic acid USP, Drug Information Digest. *American Journal of Hospital Pharmacy* 27: 494–95.

Reiss, B. S., and R. W. McLean. 1981. Drug education for providers. *American Pharmacy* NS21: 52–55.

Reuler, J. B., D. E. Girard, and D. A. Nardone. 1980. The chronic pain syndrome: Misconceptions and management. *Annals of Internal Medicine* 93: 588–96.

Rial, W. Y. 1983. Physicians frequently underutilize pain medications for terminal patients. *AMA Newsletter* 15: 1.

Rice, D. P. 1986. Demographic realities and projections of an aging population. Prepared for the 1986 Sun Valley Forum, "The role of the academic health center in dealing with the needs of an aging population," Sun Valley, Idaho, Aug. 9–14, 1986.

Rice, D. P., and C. L. Estes. 1984. Health of the elderly: Policy issues and challenges. *Health Affairs* 3: 25–49.

Rice, D. P., and J. J. Feldman. 1983. Living longer in the United States: Demographic changes and health needs of the elderly. *Milbank Memorial Fund Quarterly/ Health and Society* 61: 362–95.

Rice, D. P., and M. P. LaPlante. 1986. Chronic illness, disability, and improving longevity. Paper presented at Pew Policy Fellows Conference, May 28–30, 1986.

Richey, D. P., and A. D. Bender. 1977. Pharmacokinetic consequences of aging. *Annual Review of Pharmacology and Toxicology* 17: 49–65.

Rieger, T. 1986. Pharmacist prescribing under protocols. *California Pharmacist* 34, August 1986.

Robbins, A. S., et al. 1981. *Geriatric medicine: An education resource guide.* Cambridge, Mass.: Ballinger.

———. 1982. Studies in geriatric education: II. Educational materials and programs. *Journal of the American Geriatrics Society* 30: 340–47.

Rodeheffer, R. J., et al. 1984. Exercise cardiac output is maintained with advancing age in healthy human subjects: Cardiac dilatation and increased stroke volume compensate for a diminished heart rate. *Circulation* 69: 203–13.

Rose, C. S., et al. 1976. Age difference in Vitamin B_6 status of 617 men. *American Journal of Clinical Nutrition* 29: 847–53.

Rosen, C. E., and S. Holmes. 1978. Pharmacists' impact on chronic psychiatric outpatients in community mental health. *American Journal of Hospital Pharmacy* 35: 704–8.

Rowe, I. L. 1973. Prescriptions of psychotropic drugs by general practitioners: Two antidepressants. *Medical Journal of Australia* 1: 642–44.

Rowe, J. W. 1977. Clinical research on aging: Strategies and directions. *New England Journal of Medicine* 297: 1332–36.

———. 1985. Health care of the elderly. *New England Journal of Medicine* 312: 827–36.

Rowe, J. W., et al. 1976a. Age-adjusted standards for creatinine clearance. *Annals of Internal Medicine* 84: 567–69.

———. 1976b. The effect of age and creatinine clearance in man: A cross-sectional and longitudinal study. *Journal of Gerontology* 31: 155–63.

Rucker, T. D. 1972. The role of computers in drug utilization review. *American Journal of Hospital Pharmacy* 29: 128–33.

———. 1976. Drug information for prescribers and dispensers: Toward a model system. *Medical Care* 14: 156–65.

———. 1980. Prescription drug benefits under National Health Insurance—A blue ribbon proposal. *Pharmacy Management* 152: 23–28.

Rucker, T. D., and J. A. Visconti. 1978. *How effective are drug formularies? A descriptive and normative study.* Washington, D.C.: American Society of Hospital Pharmacists.

Rudd, P., et al. 1979. Hypertension continuation adherence. *Archives of Internal Medicine* 139: 545–49.

Ruskin, A., and C. Anello. 1980. The United States of America. In *Monitoring for drug safety*, ed. W. M. Inman, pp. 115–27. Lancaster: MTP Press.

Russell, L. B. 1981. An aging population and the use of medical care. *Medical Care* 14: 633–43.

Sackett, D. L., and R. B. Haynes. 1976. *Compliance with therapeutic regimens.* Baltimore, Md.: Johns Hopkins University Press.

Salber, E., et al. 1979. Black/white drug use in rural North Carolina. *Contemporary Pharmacy Practice* 2: 4–11.

Salerno, E. 1980. OTC medications and the elderly. *Florida Pharmacy Journal* 64: 4–9.

Schaffner, W., et al. 1983. Improving antibiotic prescribing in office practice: A controlled trial of three educational methods. *Journal of the American Medical Association* 250: 1728–32.

Schmucker, D. L. 1979. Age-related changes in drug disposition. *Pharmacological Reviews* 30: 445–56.

———. 1984. Drug disposition in the elderly: A review of critical factors. *Journal of the American Geriatrics Society* 32: 144–49.

Schneider, E. L., and J. A. Brody. 1983. Aging, natural death, and the compression of morbidity: Another view. *New England Journal of Medicine* 309: 854–56.

Schroeder, N. H., E. M. Caffey, Jr., and J. W. Lorei. 1979. Antipsychotic drugs: Can education change prescribing practices? *Journal of Clinical Psychiatry* 40: 186–89.

Schwartz, D., et al. 1962. Medication errors made by the elderly, chronically ill patients. *American Journal of Public Health* 52: 2018–29.

Schwartz, M. A. 1976. The role of the pharmacist in the patient-health team relationship. In *Patient compliance*, ed. L. Lasagna. Mount Kisco, N.Y.: Futura.

Scitovsky, A. A. 1982. Estimating the direct costs of illness. *Milbank Memorial Fund Quarterly/Health and Society* 60: 463–91.

Scitovsky, A. A., and N. M. Snyder. 1975. Medical care use by a group of fully insured aged: A case study. DHEW Pub. No. (HRA) 75-3129, U.S. Department of Health, Education, and Welfare, National Center for Health Services Research.

Seidl, L. G., et al. 1966. Studies on the epidemiology of adverse drug reactions. III. Reactions in patients on a general medical service. *Johns Hopkins Hospital Bulletin* 119: 299–315.

Seixas, F. A. 1975. Alcohol and its drug interactions. *Annals of Internal Medicine* 83: 86–92.

Sharpe, T. R. 1977. The pharmacist's potential role as a factor in increasing compliance. In *Medication compliance: A behavioral management approach*, ed. I. Barofsky, pp. 133–38. Thorofare, N.J.: Charles B. Slack.

Shaw, S. M., and L. F. Opit. 1976. Need for supervision in the elderly receiving long-term prescribed medication. *British Medical Journal* 1: 505–7.

Shepherd, A. A. M., et al. 1977. Age as a determinant of sensitivity to warfarin. *British Journal of Clinical Pharmacology* 4: 315–20.

Sherman, F. T., J. D. Warach, and L. S. Libow. 1979. Child-resistant containers for the elderly? *Journal of the American Medical Association* 241: 1001–2.

Shibaski, T., et al. 1984. Age-related changes in plasma growth hormone response to growth-hormone-releasing factor in man. *Journal of Clinical Endocrinology and Metabolism* 58: 212–14.

Shuy, R. W. 1976. The medical interview—Problems in communication. *Primary Care* 3: 365–86.

Siegel, J. S., and C. M. Taeuber. 1986. Demographic perspectives on the long-lived society. *Daedalus*, Winter 1986, pp. 77–117.

Silverman, M., and P. R. Lee. 1974. *Pills, profits, and politics*. Berkeley, Calif.: University of California Press.

Silverman, M., P. R. Lee, and M. Lydecker. 1981. *Pills and the public purse*. Berkeley, Calif.: University of California Press.

Silverman, M., and M. Lydecker, eds. 1977. *Drug coverage under national health insurance: The policy options*. DHEW Pub. No. (HRA) 77-3189, U.S. Department of Health, Education, and Welfare, National Center for Health Services Research.

Simonson, W. 1984. *Medications and the elderly: A guide for promoting proper use*. Rockville, Md.: Aspen Systems.

Simonson, W., and C. Pratt. 1982. Geriatric pharmacy curriculum in U.S.

pharmacy schools: A nationwide survey. *American Journal of Pharmaceutical Education* 46: 249–52.

Smith, C. R. 1979. Use of drugs in the aged. *Johns Hopkins Medical Journal* 145: 61–64.

Smith, M. C. 1976. Portrayal of the elderly in prescription drug advertising. *Gerontologist* 16: 329–34.

Smith, R. 1985. Doctors and the drug industry in Sweden. *British Medical Journal (Clinical Research Ed.)* 290: 448–50.

Sobel, K. G., and G. M. McCart. 1983. Drug use and accidental falls in an intermediate care facility. *Drug Intelligence and Clinical Pharmacy* 17: 539–42.

Soumerai, S. B., and J. Avorn. 1986. Economic and policy analysis of university-based drug "detailing." *Medical Care* 24: 313–31.

———. 1984. Efficacy and cost-containment in hospital pharmacotherapy: State of the art and future directions. *Milbank Memorial Fund Quarterly/Health and Society* 62: 447–74.

Soumerai, S. B., et al. 1987. Payment restrictions for prescription drugs under Medicaid: Effects on therapy, cost, and equity. *New England Journal of Medicine* 317: 550–56.

Spector, R., et al. 1978. Does intervention by a nurse improve medication compliance? *Archives of Internal Medicine* 138: 36–40.

Spence, D. L., et al. 1968. Medical student attitudes toward the geriatric patient. *Journal of the American Geriatrics Society* 16: 976–83.

Steel, K. 1978. Evaluation of the geriatric patient. In *Clinical aspects of aging*, ed. W. Reichel, pp. 3–12. Baltimore, Md.: Williams and Williams.

Steel, K., et al. 1981. Iatrogenic illness on a general medical service of a university hospital. *New England Journal of Medicine* 304: 638–42.

Stephens, R. C., C. A. Haney, and S. Underwood. 1982. Psychoactive drug use and potential misuse among persons aged 55 years and older. In *Drugs, alcohol, and aging*, eds. D. M. Petersen and F. J. Whittington, pp. 75–83. Dubuque, Iowa: Kendall/Hunt.

Stewart, R. B., W. E. Hale, and G. R. Marks. 1982. Analgesic drug use in an ambulatory elderly population. *Drug Intelligence and Clinical Pharmacy* 16: 833–36.

Stimmel, G. L., and W. F. McGhan. 1981. The pharmacist as prescriber of drug therapy: The USC pilot project. *Drug Intelligence and Clinical Pharmacy* 15: 665–72.

Stimmel, G. L., et al. 1982. Comparison of pharmacist and physician prescribing for psychiatric inpatients. *American Journal of Hospital Pharmacy* 39: 1483–86.

Stolley, P., M. Becker, and J. McEvilla. 1972. Drug prescribing and use in an American community. *Annals of Internal Medicine* 76: 537–40.

Stolley, P. D., et al. 1972. The relationship between physician characteristics and prescribing appropriateness. *Medical Care* 10: 17–28.

Strandberg, L. R., et al. 1980. Effect of comprehensive pharmaceutical services on drug use in long-term care facilities. *American Journal of Hospital Pharmacy* 37: 92–94.

Strom, B. L., K. L. Melmon, and O. S. Miettinen. 1985. Post-marketing studies of drug efficacy: Why? *American Journal of Medicine* 78: 475–80.

Svarstad, B. L. 1974. *The doctor-patient encounter: An observational study of communication and outcome.* Ph.D. dissertation, Department of Sociology, University of Wisconsin.

———. 1976. Physician-patient communication and patient conformity with medical advice. In *The growth of bureaucratic medicine: An inquiry into the dynamics of patient behavior and the organization of medical care*, ed. D. Mechanic, pp. 220–38. New York: Wiley.

———. 1983. *Patient compliance with drug regimens: An analysis of communication techniques.* Madison: School of Pharmacy, University of Wisconsin. Mimeo.

———. 1986. Patient-practitioner relationships and compliance with prescribed medical regimens. In *Application of social science to clinical medicine and health policy*, eds. L. Aiken and D. Mechanic, pp. 438–59. New Brunswick, N.J.: Rutgers University Press.

———. In press. Stress and the use of nonprescription drugs: An epidemiological study. In *Research in community and mental health*, ed. J. Greenley. Greenwich, Conn.: J.A.I. Press.

Szasz, T., and M. H. Hollender. 1956. A contribution to the philosophy of medicine: The basic models of the doctor-patient relationship. *Archives of Internal Medicine* 97: 585–92.

Takala, J., et al. 1979. Improving compliance with therapeutic regimens in hypertensive patients in a community health center. *Circulation* 59: 540–43.

Task Force on Use of Laboratory Tests in Psychiatry. 1985. Tricyclic antidepressants—Blood level measurements and clinical outcome: An APA task force report. *American Journal of Psychiatry* 142: 155–62.

Tatro, D. S., T. C. Moore, and S. N. Cohen. 1979. Computer-based system for adverse drug reaction detection and prevention. *American Journal of Hospital Pharmacy* 36: 198–201.

Tatro, D. S., et al. 1975. On-line drug interaction surveillance. *American Journal of Hospital Pharmacy* 32: 417–20.

Temin, P. 1979. Technology, regulation and market structure in the modern pharmaceutical industry. *Bell Journal of Economics* 10: 429–46.

———. 1980. *Taking your medicine: Drug regulation in the United States.* Cambridge: Harvard University Press.

Temple, R. 1983. Memorandum: Discussion paper on testing of drugs in the elderly. Food and Drug Administration, Public Health Service, U.S. Department of Health and Human Services.

———. 1985. FDA guidelines for clinical testing of drugs in the elderly.

Paper presented at Workshop on Geriatric Drug Testing and Development—Practical Applications, Bethesda, Md., Apr. 2, 1985.

Thompson, J. F., et al. 1984. Clinical pharmacists prescribing drug therapy in a geriatric setting: Outcome of a trial. *Journal of the American Geriatrics Society* 32: 154–59.

Thompson, T. L., M. G. Moran, and A. S. Nies. 1983. Psychotropic drug use in the elderly. *New England Journal of Medicine* 308: 134–37.

Trapnell, G. R. 1979. *National health insurance issues: The cost of a national prescription process.* Nutley, N.J.: Roche Laboratories.

Triggs, E. J., and R. L. Nation. 1975. Pharmacokinetics in the aged: A review. *Journal of Pharmacokinetics and Biopharmaceutics* 3: 387–418.

Triggs, E. J., et al. 1975. Pharmacokinetics in the elderly. *European Journal of Clinical Pharmacology* 8: 55–62.

Twycross, R. G. 1978. Relief of pain. In *The management of terminal disease,* ed. C. M. Saunders, Vol. 1, pp. 65–92. London: Edward Arnold.

Tyson, K. W., and J. C. Merrill. 1984. Health care institutions: Survival in a changing environment. *Journal of Medical Education* 59: 773–81.

U.S. Bureau of the Census. 1984. Census data figures. Washington, D.C.

U.S. Bureau of the Census, Economic Surveys Division. 1986. *Quarterly financial report for manufacturing, mining and trade corporations,* First Quarter. Washington, D.C.: U.S. Department of Commerce. June 1986.

U.S. Congress, Office of Technology Assessment. 1982. *Postmarketing surveillance of prescription drugs.* Washington, D.C., Nov. 1982.

———. 1984. *Technology and aging in America.* Washington, D.C., Apr. 1984.

U.S. Congress, Office of Technology Assessment. 1985. *Technology and aging in America.* OTA-BA-264. Washington, D.C., June 1985.

U.S. Congressional Budget Office. 1983. *Changing the structure of Medicare benefits: Issues and options.* Washington, D.C.: Congress of the United States.

U.S. Department of Commerce, Bureau of Economic Analysis, Interindustry Economics Division, Input Output Branch. 1984. *Detailed input-output structure of the U.S. economy 1977: Volume I. Use and make of commodities by industries, 1977.* Washington, D.C.: U.S. Department of Commerce.

U.S. Department of Health, Education, and Welfare. 1969. *Final report.* Prepared by the Task Force on Prescription Drugs. Washington, D.C.: Government Printing Office.

———. 1974. Personal out-of-pocket health expenses: United States, 1970. *Vital and Health Statistics* Series 10, No. 91 (DHEW Pub. No. HRA 74-1518). Washington, D.C.: Government Printing Office.

———. 1979. *Pharmacy and the elderly: Executive summary.* DHEW Pub. No. (HRA) 80-87.

U.S. Department of Health, Education, and Welfare; Centers for Disease

Control. 1972. *Ten-state nutrition survey, 1968–1970: III. Clinical, anthropometry, dental; IV. Biochemical; V. Dietary.* (HSM) 72-8131, 8132-33.

U.S. Department of Health, Education, and Welfare, Food and Drug Administration. 1979. *Approved drug products with proposed therapeutic equivalence evaluations.* Jan. 1979.

U.S. Department of Health, Education, and Welfare, Health Care Financing Administration. 1980. *Guide to prescription drug costs.* Apr. 1980.

U.S. Department of Health, Education, and Welfare, National Center for Health Statistics. 1969. *International comparisons of medical care utilization: A feasibility study.* Washington, D.C.: Government Printing Office.

————. 1977a. *Ambulatory medical care rendered in physicians' offices: United States, 1975.* Series 13.

————. 1977b. *Health interview survey, 1957/58–1977.* Series 10.

U.S. Department of Health, Education, and Welfare, Office of Long Term Care. 1976. *Physicians' drug prescribing patterns in skilled nursing facilities: Long-term care facility improvement campaign.* DHEW Pub. No. (PHS) 0576-50050, June 1976.

U.S. Department of Health, Education, and Welfare, Office of Nursing Home Affairs. 1976. *Assessing health care needs in skilled nursing facilities: Health professional perspectives.* Long-Term Care Facility Improvement Campaign Monograph No. 1. DHEW Pub. No. (OS) 77-50049. Rockville, Md., Mar. 1976.

U.S. Department of Health and Human Services, Health Care Financing Administration. 1981. Unpublished Medicaid statistics. Baltimore, Md.

————. 1983. *Medicare and Medicaid data book, 1983.* Publication No. HCFA 03156. Baltimore, Md., Dec. 1983.

U.S. Department of Health and Human Services, Health Care Financing Administration, Bureau of Data Management and Strategy, Office of Statistics and Data Management. 1987. *HCFA data compendium: Fiscal year 1988.* Baltimore, Md., Feb. 1987. Mimeo.

U.S. Department of Health and Human Services, Health Care Financing Administration, Medicaid Program Data Branch, Office of Research. 1983. *National Medicaid statistics: Fiscal years 1976–1982. Summary tables of state 2082's.* Baltimore, Md.

U.S. Department of Health and Human Services, Health Care Financing Administration, Office of Intergovernmental Affairs. 1985. *Medicaid services by state.* HCFA Publication No. 021558-86, Oct. 1, 1985.

U.S. Department of Health and Human Services, Health Care Financing Administration, Office of the Actuary. 1987a. *Summary of the 1987 annual reports of the Medicare Board of Trustees.* Baltimore, Md. Mimeo.

————. 1987b. *Comparison of catastrophic proposals.* Baltimore, Md. Mimeo.

U.S. Department of Health and Human Services, U.S. Public Health Service. 1984. *Gerontological nursing programs offered in the United States.* Washington, D.C.: Government Printing Office. Oct.

U.S. General Accounting Office. 1970. *Continuing problems in providing nursing home care and prescribed drugs under the Medicaid program in California.* Washington, D.C.

———. 1980. *FDA drug approval—A lengthy process that delays the availability of important new drugs.* Report to the Subcommittee on Science, Research and Technology, House Committee on Science and Technology. HRD 80-64. Washington, D.C.

U.S. House of Representatives, Select Committee on Aging. 1978. *Hearing: Poverty among America's aged.* Washington, D.C.: Government Printing Office, Aug. 9, 1978.

———. 1981. *Every ninth American.* Washington, D.C.: Government Printing Office.

———. 1984. *Background paper. The state of the elderly: The financial burden of health care.* Washington, D.C.: Government Printing Office. Jan.

U.S. House Subcommittee on Health and the Environment, Committee on Energy and Commerce. 1985. *Price increases for prescription drugs and related information.* July 15, 1985.

U.S. Senate, Special Committee on Aging. 1981. *Developments in aging: 1980, Part I.* Report No. 97-62. Washington, D.C.: Government Printing Office.

———. 1983. *Developments in aging: 1982.* Washington, D.C.: Government Printing Office.

U.S. Senate, Special Committee on Aging, Subcommittee on Long-Term Care. 1975. *Drugs in nursing homes: Misuse, costs, and kickbacks.* Supporting Paper No. 2 of *Nursing home care in the United States: Failure in public policy.* Washington, D.C.: Government Printing Office.

———. 1976. *Drugs in nursing homes: Misuse, high cost, and kickbacks.* Washington, D.C.: Government Printing Office.

Verbrugge, L. M., and F. J. Ascione. 1987. Exploring the iceberg: Common symptoms and how people care for them. *Medical Care* 25: 539–69.

Vesell, E. S. 1980. Why are toxic reactions to drugs so often undetected initially? *New England Journal of Medicine* 302: 1027–28.

Vestal, R. E. 1978. Drug use in the elderly: A review of problems and special considerations. *Drugs* 16: 358–82.

Vestal, R. E., et al. 1975. Antipyrine metabolism in man: Influence of age, alcohol, caffeine, and smoking. *Clinical Pharmacology and Therapeutics* 18: 425–32.

———. 1977. Aging and ethanol metabolism. *Clinical Pharmacology and Therapeutics* 21: 343–54.

———. 1979. Effects of age and cigarette smoking on propranolol disposition. *Clinical Pharmacology and Therapeutics* 26: 8–15.

Vladeck, B. C. 1980. *Unloving care: The nursing home tragedy.* New York: Basic Books.

Wade, A. H. *Social Security area population projections, 1985.* 1985. Actuarial

Study #95, U.S. Department of Health and Human Services, Social Security Administration, Office of the Actuary, SSA Pub. No. 11-11542, Oct. 1985.

Wadsworth, M. E. J., W. J. H. Butterfield, and R. Blaney. 1971. *Health and sickness: The choice of treatment.* London: Tavistock.

Wagner, J. L. 1982. Economic evaluations of medicines: A review of the literature. *Cost-Effectiveness of Pharmaceuticals* Report Series, Report 4. Pharmaceutical Manufacturers Association, Oct. 1982.

Waldholz, M. 1985. Prescription-drug makers aiming ad campaigns directly at public. *Wall Street Journal*, Aug. 8, 1985, p. 23.

Waldo, D. R. 1987. Outpatient prescription drug spending by the Medicare population. *Health Care Financing Review* 9, Fall 1987, pp. 83–89.

Waldo, D. R., and H. C. Lazenby. 1984. Demographic characteristics and health care use and expenditures by the aged in the United States: 1977–1984. *Health Care Financing Review* 6, Fall 1984, pp. 1–29.

Wallace, S., B. Whiting, and J. Runcie. 1976. Factors affecting drug binding in plasma of elderly patients. *British Journal of Clinical Pharmacology* 3: 327–30.

Wandless, I., and J. W. Davie. 1977. Can drug compliance in the elderly be improved? *British Medical Journal* 1: 359–61.

Wardell, W. M., J. DiRaddo, and A. G. Trimble. 1980. Development of new drugs originated and acquired by United States-owned pharmaceutical firms, 1963–1976. *Clinical Pharmacology and Therapeutics* 28: 270–77.

Wardell, W. M., M. S. May, and A. G. Trimble. 1981. Recent trends in United States drug development, 1977–1979. Abstract. *Clinical Pharmacology and Therapeutics* 29: 288.

Waxman, H. M., M. Klein, and E. A. Carner. 1985. Drug misuse in nursing homes: An institutional addiction? *Hospital and Community Psychiatry* 36: 886–87.

Weintraub, M. 1976. Intelligent noncompliance and capricious compliance. In *Patient compliance*, ed. L. Lasagna, Vol. X, pp. 39–47. Mt. Kisco, N.Y.: Futura.

Weintraub, M., W. Au, and L. Lasagna. 1973. Compliance as a determinant of serum digoxin concentration. *Journal of the American Medical Association* 224: 481–85.

Weisbrod, B. A., and J. H. Huston. 1983. Benefits and costs of human vaccines in developed countries: An evaluative survey. *Cost-Effectiveness of Pharmaceuticals* Report Series, Report 2. Pharmaceutical Manufacturers Association, July 1983.

White, K. L., T. F. Williams, and B. G. Greenberg. 1961. The ecology of medical care. *New England Journal of Medicine* 265: 885.

Whiting, B., I. Wandless, and D. J. Sumner. 1978. A computer-assisted review of digoxin therapy in the elderly. *British Heart Journal* 40: 8–13.

Whittington, F. J., et al. 1982. Sex differences in prescription drug use of older adults. In *Drugs, alcohol, and aging*, eds. D. M. Petersen and F. J. Whittington, pp. 65–73. Dubuque, Iowa: Kendall/Hunt.

Wilber, J. A., and J. G. Barrow. 1969. Reducing elevated blood pressure: experience found in a community. *Minnesota Medicine* 52: 1303–6.

Wilensky, G. R. 1981. Government and the financing of health care. Paper presented to American Economic Association meetings, Washington, D.C., Dec. 1981. (Also found in Papers and Proceedings Issue of the *American Economic Review*, May 1982.)

———. 1983. Statement before the Special Committee on Aging, U.S. Senate, Apr. 13, 1983.

Williams, T. F. 1986. Current status of biomedical and behavioral research in aging. Paper presented at Sun Valley Forum on Nation's Health, Sun Valley, Idaho, Aug. 10, 1986.

Williams, T. F., et al. 1973. Appropriate placement of the chronically ill aged—A successful approach by evaluation. *Journal of the American Medical Association* 226: 1332–35.

Williams, W. 1985. Glory days end for pharmaceuticals. *New York Times*, Feb. 24, 1985, p. 1.

Williamson, J. 1979. Adverse reactions to prescribed drugs in the elderly. In *Drugs and the elderly*, eds. J. Crooks and I. H. Stevenson, pp. 239–46. Baltimore, Md.: University Park Press.

Wilson, P. A. 1983. Hospital use by the aging population. *Inquiry* 18: 332–44.

World Health Organization, Regional Office for Europe. 1985. *Drugs for the elderly*. Copenhagen, Denmark.

Wynne, R. D., and F. Heller. 1973. Drug overuse among the elderly: A growing problem. *Perspectives on Aging* 11: 15–18.

Yesalis, C. E., III, D. P. Lipson, G. J. Norwood, et al. 1984. Capitation payment for pharmacy services: I. Impact on drug use and pharmacist dispensing behavior. *Medical Care* 22: 737–45.

Yesalis, C. E., III, G. J. Norwood, and D. K. Helling. 1984. Capitation payment for pharmacy services: II. Impact on costs. *Medical Care* 22: 746–54.

Yesalis, C. E., III, G. J. Norwood, D. P. Lipson, et al. 1981. Use and costs under the Iowa capitation drug program. *Health Care Financing Review* 3, Fall 1981, pp. 127–36.

Yosselson, S. 1976. Drugs and nutrition. *Drug Intelligence and Clinical Pharmacy* 10: 8–14.

Zawadski, R. T., G. B. Glazer, and E. Lurie. 1978. Psychotropic drug use among institutionalized and noninstitutionalized Medicaid aged in California. *Journal of Gerontology* 33: 825–34.

Index

Library of Congress Cataloging-in-Publication Data

Lipton, Helene L.
  Drugs and the elderly.

  Bibliography: p.
  Includes index.
    1. Aged—United States—Drug use.   2. Medication
abuse—United States.   3. Drug abuse—United States
—Prevention.   I. Lee, Philip R.   II. Title.
HV5824.A33L56 1988   362.2'9   87-33574
ISBN 0-8047-1295-6 (alk. paper)

Printed and bound by CPI Group (UK) Ltd, Croydon, CR0 4YY

16/04/2025

14658401-0001